100 Dumbbell Workouts

2023

N. Rey | darebee.com

First Printing, 2023.
ISBN 10: 1-84481-182-4
ISBN 13: 978-1-84481-182-3
Published by New Line Books, London

Warning and Disclaimer
Although every precaution has been taken to verify the accuracy of the information contained
herein, the author and publisher assume no responsibility for any errors or omissions. No liability
is assumed for damage or injury that may result from the use of information contained within.

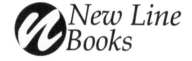

Author Bio

Neila Rey is the founder of Darebee, a global fitness resource. She is committed to democratizing fitness by removing the barriers to it and increasing accessibility. Every workout published in her books utilizes the latest in exercise science and has undergone thorough field testing and refinement through Darebee volunteers. When she's not busy running Darebee she is focused on finding fresh ways to make exercise easier and more enjoyable.

Thank you!

Thank you for purchasing **100 Dumbbell Workouts**, DAREBEE project print edition. DAREBEE is a non-profit global fitness resource dedicated to making fitness accessible for everyone, no matter their circumstances. The project is supported exclusively via user donations and paperback royalties.

After printing costs and store fees every book developed by the DAREBEE project makes $1 and it goes directly into our project maintenance and development fund.

Each sale helps us keep the DAREBEE resource growing, maintain it and keep it up. Thank you for making a difference in its future!

Other books in this series include:

100 No-Equipment Workouts Vol 1.
100 No-Equipment Workouts Vol 2.
100 No-Equipment Workouts Vol 3.
100 No-Equipment Workouts Vol 4.
100 Office Workouts
Pocket Workouts: 100 no-equipment workouts
ABS 100 Workouts: Visual Easy-To-Follow ABS Exercise Routines for All Fitness Levels
100 HIIT Workouts: Visual easy-to-follow routines for all fitness levels

100 dumbbell workouts

1. Agent Of Chaos
2. Armory Plus
3. Arm Shred
4. Back & Biceps Express
5. Back & Biceps
6. Because I Can
7. Benched
8. Berserk: Guts
9. Bicep & Triceps
10. Big Back
11. Bigger Arms
12. Body Patch Plus
13. Brute Abs
14. Brute Arms & Back
15. Brute Legday
16. Buff
17. Bulk Order
18. Butcher
19. Catalyst
20. Chest & Back
21. Come Back Stronger
22. Cultivator
23. Digger
24. Dumbbell Abs
25. Dynamic Dumbbell
26. Endgame Plus
27. Enemy Lines Plus
28. Epic Arms
29. Epic Gains
30. Farmer
31. Full Body Built
32. Fullbody Render Plus
33. Gainer
34. Glutes Sculpt
35. Goliath
36. Hammer
37. Hardgainer
38. HD Arms
39. Heavy Duty
40. Hephaestus
41. Home Upperbody Tone
42. Hunter Plus
43. Hybrid
44. Iron Dragon
45. Ironheart
46. Iron Will
47. Jacked
48. Jungle
49. Lift & Tone
50. Like A Boss
51. Mammoth
52. Mason Plus
53. Mave
54. Meta Burn
55. Moving Mountains
56. Muscle Factory Lowerbody
57. Muscle Factory Upperbody
58. Ox
59. Pixie
60. Power 10
61. Power 18
62. Power 20
63. Power 25
64. Power Circuit Plus
65. Power HIIT
66. Power Pump
67. Power Row
68. PPL Legs A
69. PPL Legs B
70. PPL Pull A
71. PPL Pull B
72. PPL Push A
73. PPL Push B
74. Pure Power
75. Recomp
76. Renegade
77. Rise & Grind
78. Sentinel Plus
79. Serious Lifts
80. Shredder Plus
81. Smiter
82. Steelworks Plus
83. Strength & Power
84. Strong & Beautiful
85. Stuntman
86. Superhero Strength Plus
87. Super Strength
88. Threshold
89. Trim & Tone Arms
90. Tyr
91. Under Construction
92. Upperbody Blast
93. Upperbody Builder
94. Upperbody Forge
95. Upperbody Tendon Strength Plus
96. Upper Body Sculpt
97. Valour
98. V-Taper
99. Work Of Art
100. XXL Biceps

How To Choose The Right
Dumbbell Weight

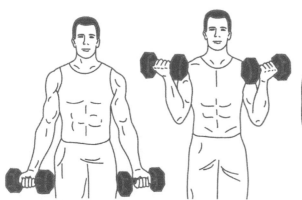

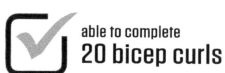

✓ able to complete
20 bicep curls

men   ~ 15-17lb (7-8kg)
women ~ 11-13lb (5-6kg)

Adjustable
Saves space

Comfortable Grip
Durable

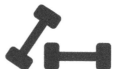

Light
Perfect for punches

Monitor how many sets and reps you can do continuously and, if you find
that you can do more than your target number of repetitions, increase the amount of weight
you're lifting by 1-2 pounds (0.5-1kg).

Don't settle for just one set of dumbbells. Ensure you have a range of different weights
to accommodate the various exercises you want to perform.

How To Choose Dumbbells

Dumbbells are a steady load that is external to the body. They can bring about great adaptations to the muscles increasing their strength, power and endurance precisely because of that. However, because the load is external to the body it presents a very-near constant load to joints and tendons. As a result it can lead to injury much faster than say, doing bodyweight exercises.

To avoid these you need to focus on two things: First, technique. It's important you use proper technique when lifting weights. So if you were to do, for instance, bicep curls with your dumbbells it's super-important to maintain great form and actually lift with the bicep and shoulder muscles, primarily and not use your entire body to 'swing' the dumbbell up to your shoulder as you perform the curl.

The second thing to focus on is the weight you lift. For dumbbells and general dumbbell lifting exercises that target the biceps, triceps and shoulders the rule of thumb is to use a set of two 5 – 10 lbs weights (approx. 2 – 5 kgs) for women and 10 – 20 lbs weights (approx. 5 – 10kgs) for men.

If you have made that choice and storage is an issue, then volume can always be substituted for weight when it comes to progressing your dumbbell strength training at home. If you started out with 20 lbs dumbbells and you have outgrown them, you could, for instance, do 20 consecutive curls with 20 lbs dumbbell weights instead of doing ten with higher weight dumbbells which you haven't got. Scientific analysis of the results shows that in terms of strength attained and size of the muscles this is a good substitute that delivers virtually identical results to lifting heavier with fewer repetitions.

SAMPLE CIRCUIT WORKOUT

LEVEL I 3 sets **LEVEL II** 5 sets **LEVEL III** 7 sets **REST** up to 2 minutes

10 jumping jack

20 high knees

40 side-to-side chops

one squat

20 lunges

10-count plank hold

20 climbers

10 plank jump-ins

to failure push-ups

Difficulty Levels:

Level I: normal
Level II: hard
Level III: advanced

Repeat the circuit (all exercises)
3, 5 or 7 times in total depending on
the level you choose

1 set

10 jumping jacks
20 high knees (10 each leg)
40 side-to-side chops (20 each side)
one squat = 1 squat
20 lunges (10 each leg)
10-count plank (hold while counting to 10)
20 climbers (10 each leg)
10 plank jump-ins
to failure push-ups (your maximum)

Up to 2 minutes rest between sets
30 seconds, 60 seconds or 2 minutes -
it's up to you.

SAMPLE CLASSIC WORKOUT

2 minutes rest between exercises

20 push-ups **x 4 sets** in total
20 seconds rest between sets

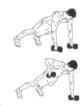
10 renegade rows **x 4 sets** in total
20 seconds rest between sets

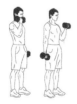
20 alt bicep curls **x 4 sets** in total
20 seconds rest between sets

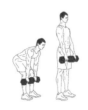
10 deadlifts **x 4 sets** in total
20 seconds rest between sets

Complete all sets for each exercise first,
then move on to the next exercise:

E.g., Do 20 push-ups, rest 20 seconds
then repeat - 4 times in total.
Move on to renegade rows and so on.

All reps are given in total:

E.g., 10 renegade rows = 5 reps per side.

2 minutes rest between exercises

30 seconds, 60 seconds or 2 minutes -
it's up to you.

Instructions

The workout posters are read from left to right.

There are two primary types of DAREBEE workouts: circuit and classic. Circuit workouts have levels I, II and III with levels and sets located at the top of the poster. The entire poster is one single set. Complete all of the exercises and their corresponding reps before taking a break. You then rest and repeat until you've done all of the sets for your level. Classic workouts have sets and rest times listed under each exercise. You complete all sets for every exercise first and then move on to the next exercise in a classic setup.

"Reps" stands for repetitions, how many times an exercise is performed. Reps are usually located next to each exercise's name. Number of reps is always a total number for both legs / arms / sides. It's easier to count this way: e.g. if it says 20 climbers, it means that both legs are already counted in - it is 10 reps each leg.

Reps *to failure* or *maximum* reps means to muscle failure = your personal maximum, you repeat the move until you can't do it properly anymore. It can be anything from one rep to twenty, normally applies to more challenging exercises. The goal is to do as many repetitions as you possibly can.

The transition from exercise to exercise is an important part of each circuit (set) - it is often what makes a particular workout more effective. Transitions are carefully worked out to hyperload specific muscle groups more for better results. For example if you see a plank followed by push-ups it means that you start performing push-ups right after you finished with the plank avoiding dropping your body on the floor in between.

If you can't do all out push-ups yet on Level I it is perfectly acceptable to do knee push-ups instead. The modification works the same muscles as a full push-up but lowers the load significantly helping you build up on it first. It is also ok to switch to knee push-ups at any point if you can no longer do full push-ups in the following sets.

Video Exercise Library: http://darebee.com/exercises

The workouts are organized in alphabetical order so you can find the workouts you favor easier and faster.

Use one of the following training plans to create a training routine that suits you best:

Gladiator

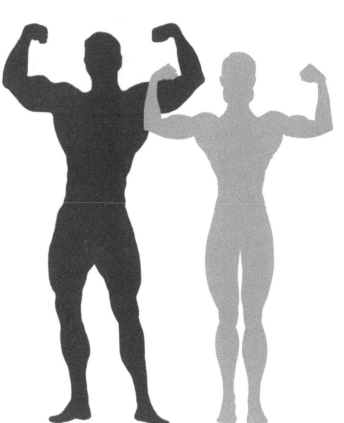

Day 1	**Fullbody Workout**
Day 2	**Rest** or casual training
Day 3	**Upperbody Workout**
Day 4	**Lowerbody Workout**
Day 5	**Rest** or casual training
Day 6	**Fullbody Workout**
Day 7	**Rest** or casual training

Knight

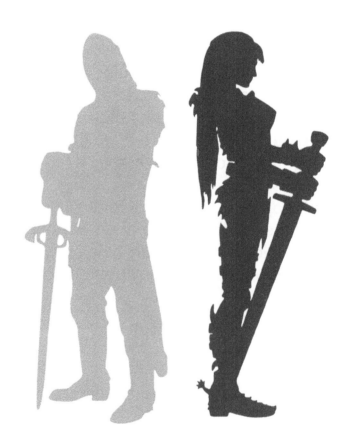

Day 1	**Fullbody Workout**
Day 2	**Rest** or casual training
Day 3	**Fullbody Workout**
Day 4	**Rest** or casual training
Day 5	**Fullbody Workout**
Day 6	**Rest** or casual training
Day 7	**Rest** or casual training

PUSH
PULL
LEGS
PPL

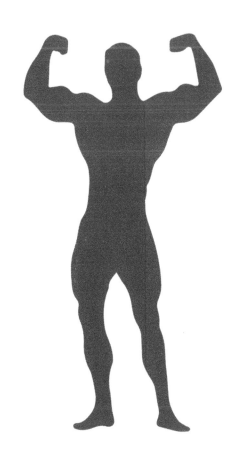

Day 1	**Push** Workout (A or B)
Day 2	**Rest** or casual training
Day 3	**Pull** Workout (A or B)
Day 4	**Rest** or casual training
Day 5	**Legs** Workout (A or B)
Day 6	**Rest** or casual training
Day 7	**Rest** or casual training

Guardian

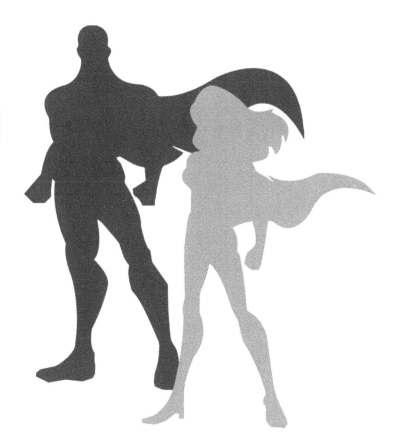

Day 1	**Fullbody** Workout
Day 2	**Rest** or casual training
Day 3	**Any type of cardio**
Day 4	**Rest** or casual training
Day 5	**Fullbody** Workout
Day 6	**Rest** or casual training
Day 7	**Rest** or casual training

Amazon

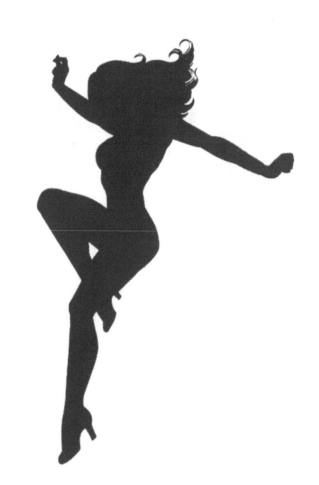

Day 1 **Fullbody Workout**

Day 2 **Rest** or casual training

Day 3 **Any type of cardio**

Day 4 **Rest** or casual training

Day 5 **Fullbody Workout**

Day 6 **Rest** or casual training

Day 7 **Any type of cardio**

Viking

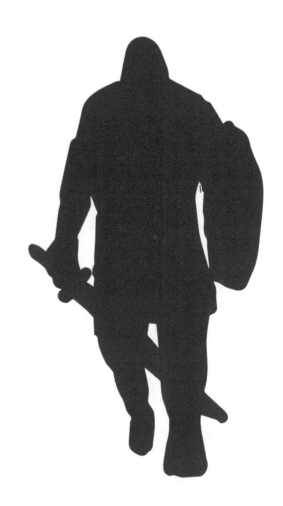

Day 1 **Lowerbody Workout**

Day 2 **Rest** or casual training

Day 3 **Upperbody Workout**

Day 4 **Rest** or casual training

Day 5 **Lowerbody Workout**

Day 6 **Upperbody Workout**

Day 7 **Rest** or casual training

Spartan

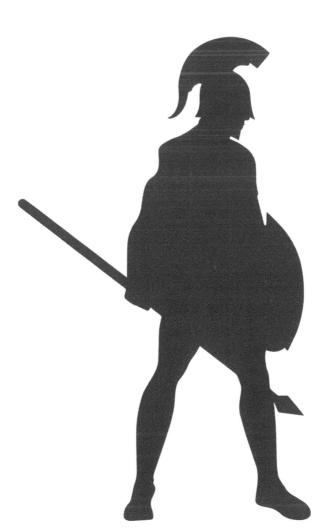

Day 1   **Fullbody Workout**

Day 2   **Rest** or casual training

Day 3   **Fullbody Workout**

Day 4   **Rest** or casual training

Day 5   **Upperbody Workout**

Day 6   **Lowerbody Workout**

Day 7   **Rest** or casual training

Valkyrie

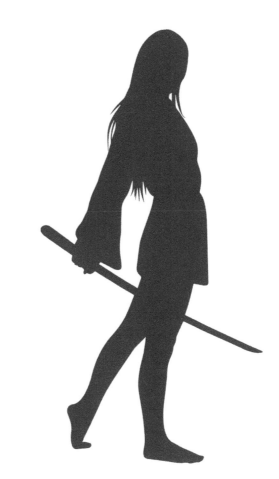

Day 1   **Lowerbody Workout**

Day 2   **Upperbody Workout**

Day 3   **Rest** or casual training

Day 4   **Rest** or casual training

Day 5   **Fullbody Workout**

Day 6   **Rest** or casual training

Day 7   **Rest** or casual training

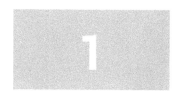 # Agent Of Chaos

As the name suggests, Agent Of Chaos, is a workout that mixes things up a little. Combining bodyweight exercises with dumbbells it forces your body to undergo a stronger adaptation response for greater fitness gains in shorter time.

Type: Circuit
What It Works:

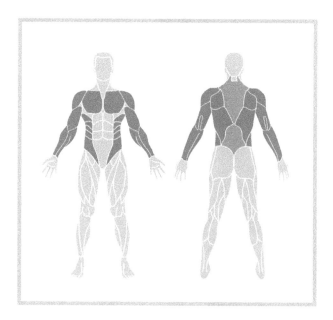

AGENT of CHAOS

DAREBEE WORKOUT © darebee.com

LEVEL I 3 sets **LEVEL II** 4 sets **LEVEL III** 5 sets **REST** up to 2 minutes

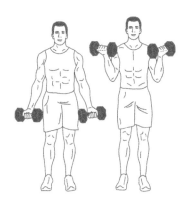

8 bicep curls

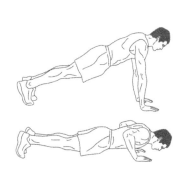

4 push-ups

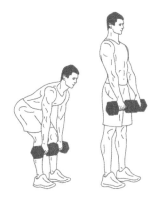

8 deadlifts

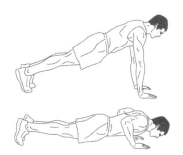

4 push-ups

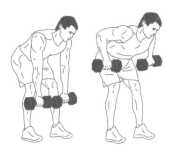

8 bent over rows

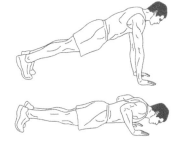

4 push-ups

2   Armory Plus

Armory Plus is a full body, light-weights workout that targets fascial fitness to produce extra power and explosiveness in every move you make. The moves are designed to force muscles to work in a precise way through upper body combat moves and as fatigue begins to kick in, you find yourself in the sweat zone, using your entire body as a primary weapon.

Type: Circuit
What It Works:

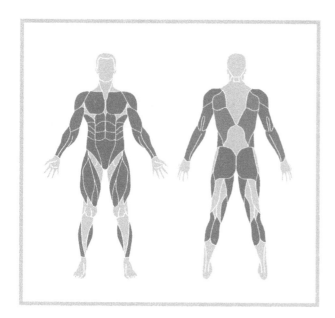

ARMORY+

DAREBEE WORKOUT © darebee.com

LEVEL I 3 sets **LEVEL II** 5 sets **LEVEL III** 7 sets **REST** up to 2 minutes

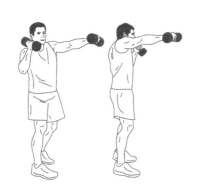

30 punches

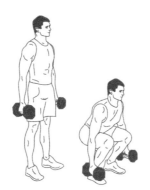

10 squats

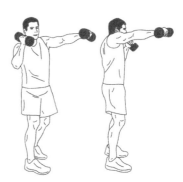

30 punches

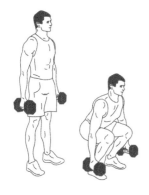

10 squats

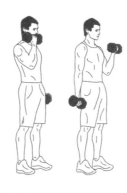

30 bicep curls

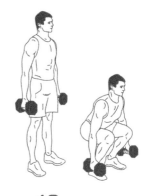

10 squats

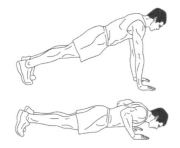

10 push-ups

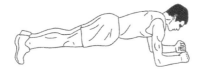

30-count elbow plank

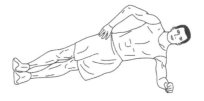

30-count side plank

3　Arm Shred

Arm Shred lives up to both its premise and promise with an upper body strength routine that focuses on developing quality muscle through successive loads as you go from set to set. Your arms will probably be a little sore the following day but your overall strength rating will go up.

Type: Classic
What It Works:

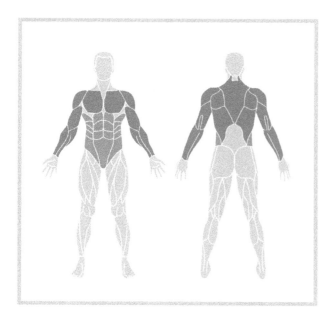

ARM SHRED

DAREBEE
WORKOUT
© darebee.com
60 seconds rest
between exercises

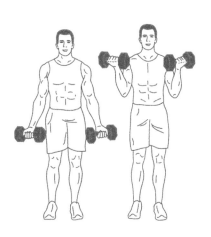

bicep curls
12 / 10 / 8 / 6 reps
30 seconds rest
between sets

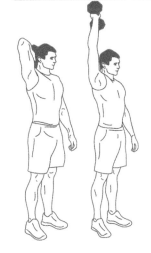

tricep extensions
6 / 5 / 4 / 3 reps per side
30 seconds rest
between sets

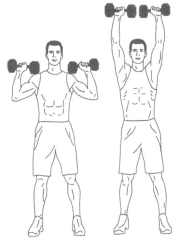

shoulder press
12 / 10 / 8 / 6 reps
30 seconds rest
between sets

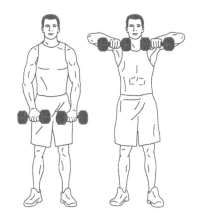

upright rows
12 / 10 / 8 / 6 reps
30 seconds rest between sets

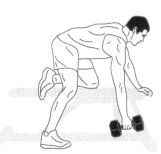
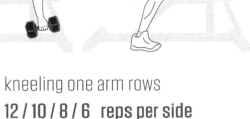

kneeling one arm rows
12 / 10 / 8 / 6 reps per side
30 seconds rest between sets

4   Back & Biceps Express

If you have some weights that challenge you handy the Back and Biceps Express workout is an easy fit into almost every challenging schedule. It targets precisely the muscles of the upper body.

Type: Classic
What It Works:

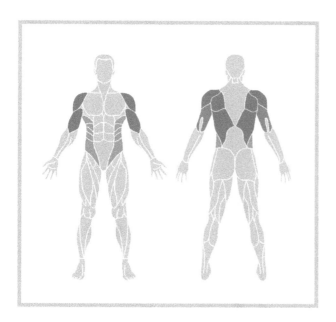

BACK & BICEPS

DAREBEE WORKOUT

© darebee.com

EXPRESS

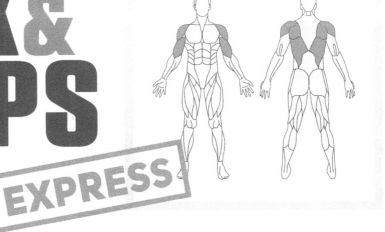

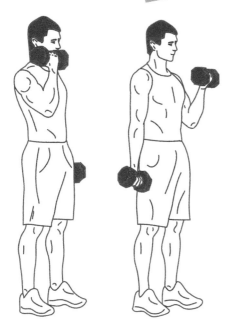

20 alternating bicep curls
x 4 sets in total
20 seconds rest
between sets

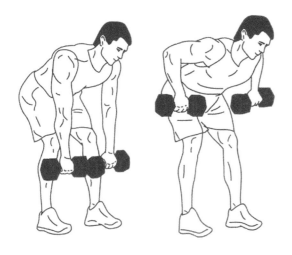

10 bent over rows
x 4 sets in total
20 seconds rest
between sets

5 Back & Biceps

Upper body strength is expressed, primarily, through the strength in our arms and the muscles on our back. The Back and Biceps workout uses barbells for a targeted workout on a critical muscle group.

Type: Classic
What It Works:

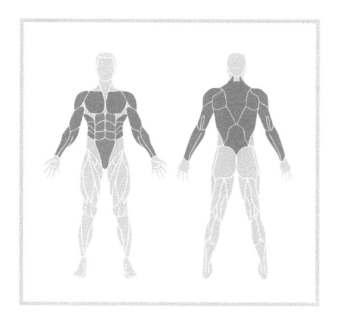

BACK & BICEPS

DAREBEE WORKOUT
© darebee.com

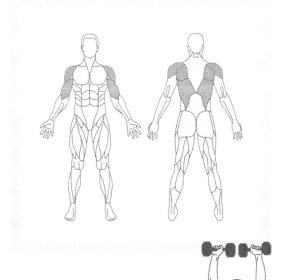

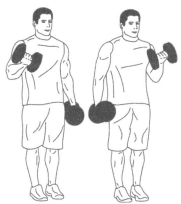

10 alt bicep curls
x 3 sets in total
20 seconds rest
between sets

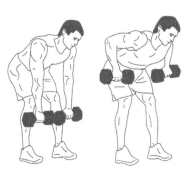

8 bent over rows
x 3 sets in total
20 seconds rest
between sets

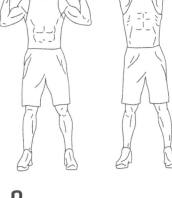

8 shoulder press
x 3 sets in total
20 seconds rest
between sets

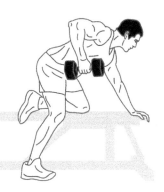

16 kneeling one arm rows
x 3 sets in total
20 seconds rest between sets

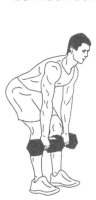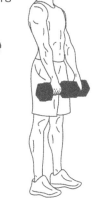

8 dead lifts
x 3 sets in total
20 seconds rest between sets

6   Because I Can

Because I Can is a dumbbells based home workout that uses compound moves to move muscles along the body's kinetic chain. It appears to be deceptively easy but it makes a considerable oxygen demand so it strengthens your cardiovascular system while helping you become stronger and feel more in control of your body.

Type: Circuit
What It Works:

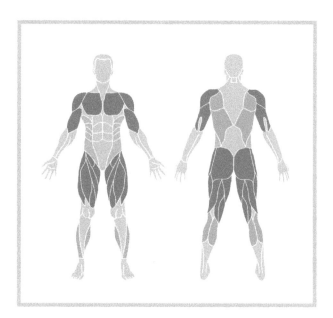

BECAUSE I CAN

DAREBEE WORKOUT © darebee.com

LEVEL I 3 sets **LEVEL II** 4 sets **LEVEL III** 5 sets **REST** up to 2 minutes

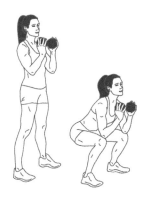

12 goblet squats

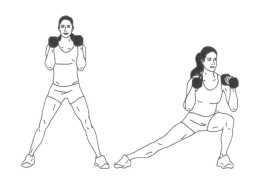

12 side lunges

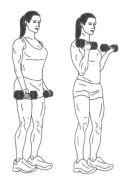

12 bicep curls

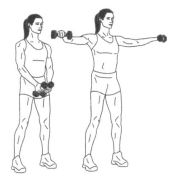

6 lateral raises

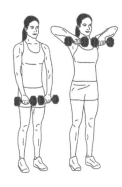

6 upright rows

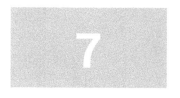

Benched

If you have a set of dumbells and a bench (or at least something that could double as one) you've got yourself a strength workout that will trigger adaptive pressures in all the major, upper body muscle groups. Make this a go-to workout whenever you're looking to build upper body strength and enjoy the benefits.

Type: Classic
What It Works:

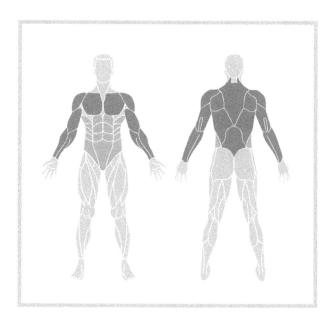

BENCHED

DAREBEE WORKOUT © darebee.com

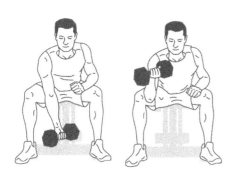
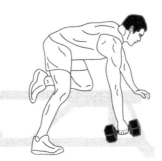

10 / 10 bicep curls
x 4 sets in total | 20 seconds rest

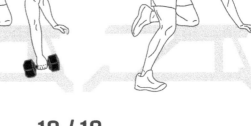

10 / 10 rows
x 4 sets in total | 20 seconds rest

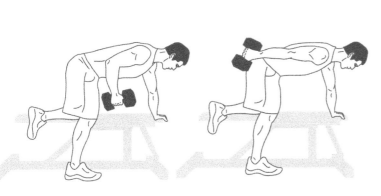

10 / 10 tricep extensions
x 4 sets in total | 20 seconds rest

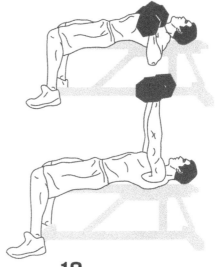

10 chest press
x 4 sets in total | 20 seconds rest

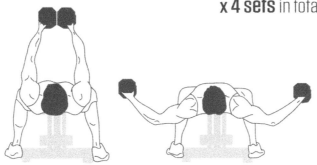

10 chest fly **x 4 sets** in total | 20 seconds rest

8 Berserk: Guts

Add something extra in your training routine, a deeper dimension that taps into your secret source of power, the thing that makes you go incandescent when you have to face an Apostle. No self-respecting Merc, former member of the Band of the Hawk can accept to be anything than the very best, when it comes to physical training. The Guts workout will make sure that when it comes to wielding the Dragonslayer, your body will be more than just up to it.

Type: Circuit
What It Works:

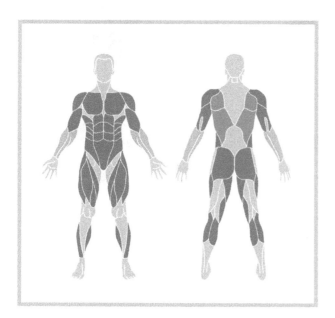

GUTS

DAREBEE WORKOUT © darebee.com

100 reps in total each exercise | split into manageable sets

Level I throughout the day **Level II** repeat once **Level III** twice in one day

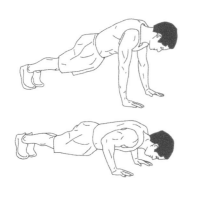

push-ups

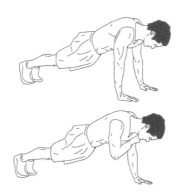

shoulder taps

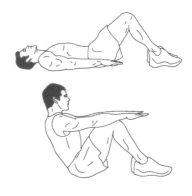

sit-ups

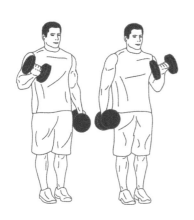

bicep curls

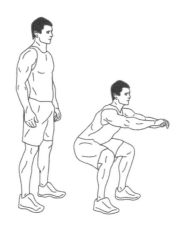

squats

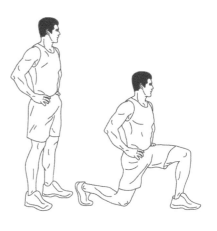

lunges

9   Bicep & Triceps

Upper body strength is what makes us capable of throwing balls faster, swinging rackets harder, throwing punches with more power and carrying shopping bags without feeling we need a pit stop. Biceps and triceps are a large component of upper body strength. As you'd expect the Biceps & Triceps workout lives up to its name by working out biceps and triceps. 'Nuff said.

Type: Classic
What It Works:

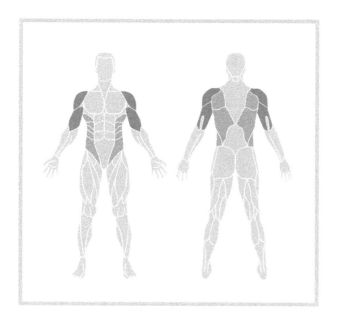

biceps & triceps

DAREBEE WORKOUT © darebee.com

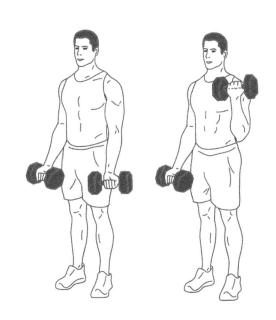

20 bicep curls
x 3 sets in total
30 seconds rest
between sets

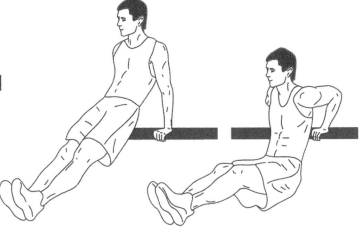

20 tricep dips
x 3 sets in total
30 seconds rest
between sets

10 Big Back

Just because they're behind us and we don't see them, doesn't mean that back muscles are not important. Acting like levers and pulleys in the skeleton, back muscles are key to powering the upper and power body through dynamic and static movements. That means that they can often play a key role to increasing power. The Big Back workout works out this very important muscle group so when you feel the need for power your back muscles can back it up.

Type: Classic
What It Works:

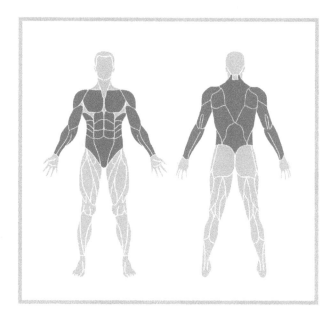

BIG BACK

DAREBEE WORKOUT © darebee.com

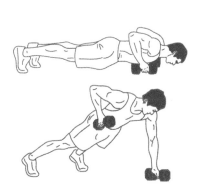

12 push-up renegade rows
x **4 sets** in total
20 seconds rest

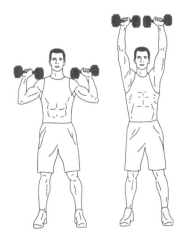

8 shoulder press
x **4 sets** in total
20 seconds rest

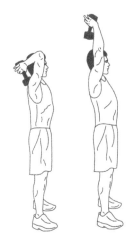

8 tricep extensions
x **4 sets** in total
20 seconds rest

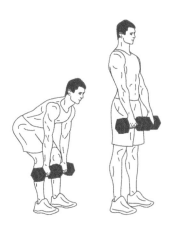

8 deadlifts
x **4 sets** in total
20 seconds rest

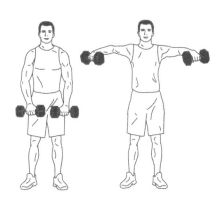

8 lateral raises
x **4 sets** in total
20 seconds rest

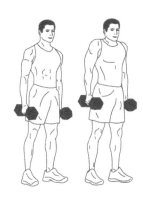

12 shrugs
x **4 sets** in total
20 seconds rest

 # Bigger Arms

Bigger Arms is a dumbbells workout that's designed to activate the body's adaptive response and give you stronger, bigger arms. Because muscles are an organ it will also help you feel healthier and more alive and it will give you a greater sense of freedom of your body and of your life.

Type: Classic
What It Works:

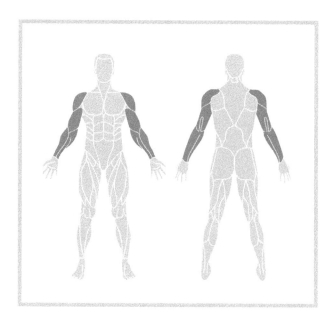

BIGGER ARMS

DAREBEE WORKOUT © darebee.com
2 minutes rest between exercises

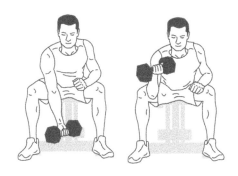

8 / 8 bicep curls **x 5 sets** in total
60 seconds rest between sets

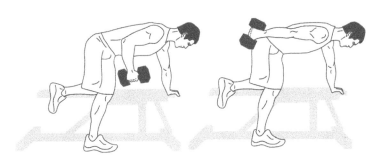

8 / 8 tricep extensions **x 5 sets** in total
60 seconds rest between sets

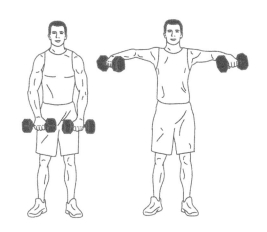

8 lateral raises **x 5 sets** in total
20 seconds rest between sets

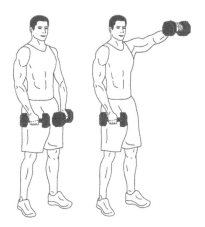

8 / 8 forward raises **x 5 sets** in total
20 seconds rest between sets

12 Body Patch Plus

Body Patch+ is a full bodyweight high-performance workout that is designed to help you develop strength, core stability and dense, powerful muscles. The exercises are performed in their fullest range of movement with punches utilizing full body movement behind them for extra strength and power. You will need two sets of weights. A heavy set for lunges and push-up shoulder taps (usually between 10-15 kgs) and a light one for punches (usually between 1- 3 kg). The load on the muscles is designed to activate contractile muscle tissue growth and create more neurons per muscle fiber resulting in greater strength and speed.

Type: Circuit
What It Works:

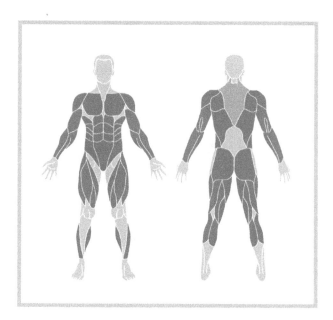

BODY PATCH+

DAREBEE WORKOUT
ⓒ darebee.com
LEVEL I 3 sets
LEVEL II 5 sets
LEVEL III 7 sets
REST up to 2 minutes

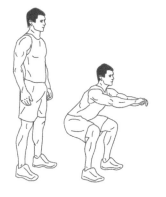

40 squats

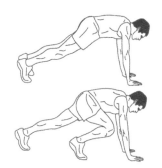

40 slow climbers

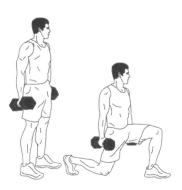

20 lunges

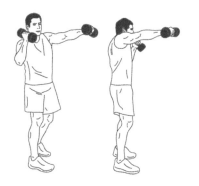

40 punches

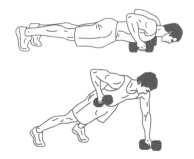

20 push-up + renegade row

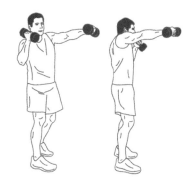

40 punches

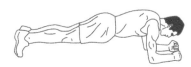

20-count plank

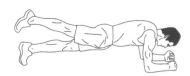

20-count raised leg plank

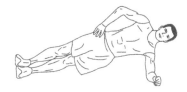

20-count side plank

13 Brute Abs

Because the abdominal muscle group is already pretty strong, eliciting an adaptation response from it requires a lot of extra effort. Enter Brute Abs. This is a workout designed to do just that. If you have a handy dumbbell you can load your abs to elicit the adaptation response, increase their strength and maybe, even, their size. Be slow, methodical and controlled in your execution here and the workout will reward you.

Type: Classic
What It Works:

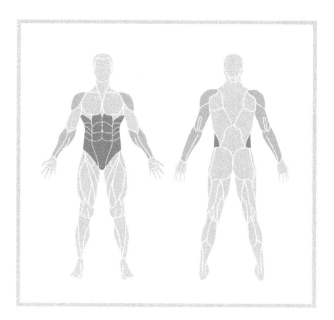

BRUTE

DAREBEE WORKOUT © darebee.com 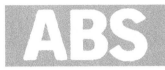 **ABS**

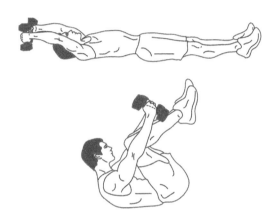

10 sit-up folds
x 4 sets in total
20 seconds rest between sets

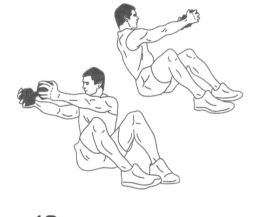

10 sitting twists
x 4 sets in total
20 seconds rest between sets

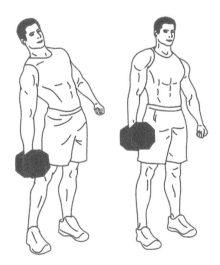

10 side tilts
x 4 sets in total
20 seconds rest between sets

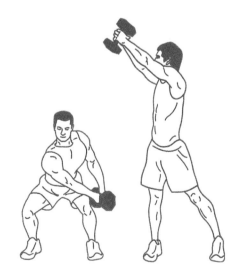

10 cross chops
x 4 sets in total
20 seconds rest between sets

14   Brute Arms & Back

Weights are extrinsic which means they present the body with a steady load throughout the workout. This can activate adaptation faster and can lead to quicker gains in strength and muscle growth, particularly for men. Women also benefit from weight training. Lacking the same testosterone levels as men, they usually experience gains in firmness and improved upper body muscle tone.

Type: Classic
What It Works:

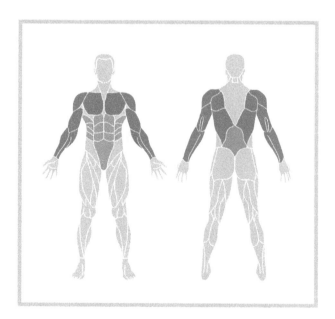

BRUTE

DAREBEE WORKOUT © darebee.com **ARMS & BACK**

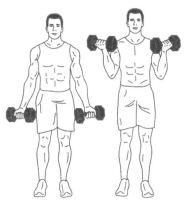

12 bicep curls
x 4 sets in total
20 seconds rest
between sets

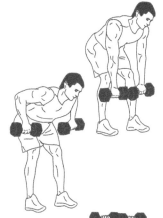

12 bent over rows
x 4 sets in total
20 seconds rest
between sets

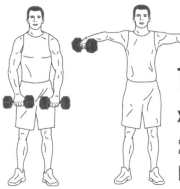

12 lateral raises
x 4 sets in total
20 seconds rest
between sets

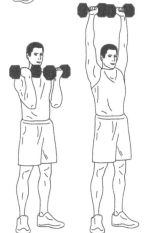

12 arnold press
x 4 sets in total
20 seconds rest
between sets

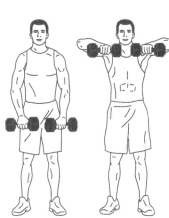

12 upright tows
x 4 sets in total
20 seconds rest
between sets

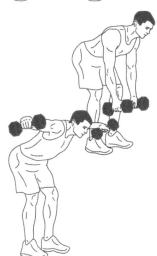

12 bent over raises
x 4 sets in total
20 seconds rest
between sets

15 Brute Legday

If you have a pair of dumbbells lying around the Brute Leg Day workout will add the extrinsic weight you need to take your strength workout to a new level altogether. Strength workouts help increase overall performance by affecting muscle density and helping increase the size of muscles.

Type: Classic
What It Works:

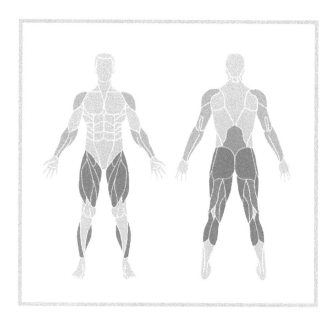

BRUTE

DAREBEE WORKOUT © darebee.com   **LEG DAY**

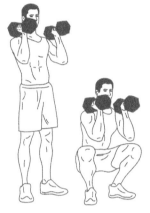

10 squats
x 4 sets in total
20 seconds rest between sets

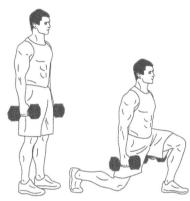

10 lunges
x 4 sets in total
20 seconds rest between sets

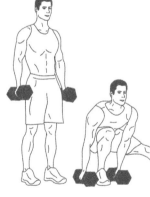

10 side lunges
x 4 sets in total
20 seconds rest between sets

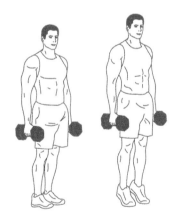

20 calf raises
x 3 sets in total
20 seconds rest between sets

10 single leg straight leg dead lifts
x 4 sets in total
20 seconds rest between sets

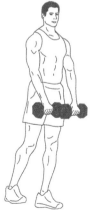
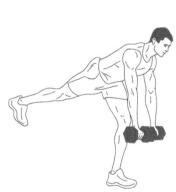

16 Buff

Resistance training enables the body to experience a higher load in a targeted muscle-group way. As a result the adaptive response this elicits leads to greater strength and larger muscle size. Which means that Buff is a difficulty Level 5 workout and not suitable if you're new to all this. For everyone else however this has to be that occasional workout you go to in order to test how far you've got on your fitness journey.

Type: Classic
What It Works:

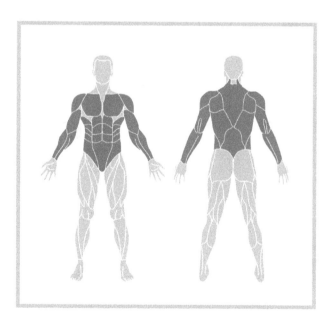

BUFF

DAREBEE WORKOUT © darebee.com

2 minutes rest between exercises

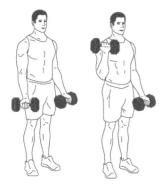

10 bicep curls
x 5 sets in total
60 seconds rest
between sets

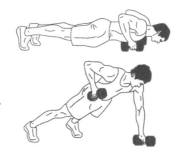

10 renegade row
push-ups
x 5 sets in total
60 seconds rest
between sets

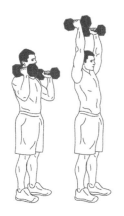

10 shoulder press
x 5 sets in total
60 seconds rest
between sets

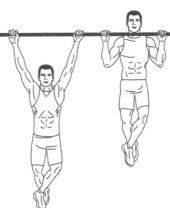

to failure
pull-ups
x 5 sets in total
60 seconds rest
between sets

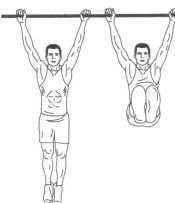

to failure
leg raises
x 5 sets in total
60 seconds rest
between sets

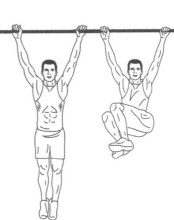

to failure
knee-up & twists
x 5 sets in total
60 seconds rest
between sets

 # Bulk Order

Bulk Order is a strength workout that will help you trigger the body's adaptation response and build stronger muscles. Strong muscles create strong bones and strong bones make for a strong and healthy brain.

Type: Classic
What It Works:

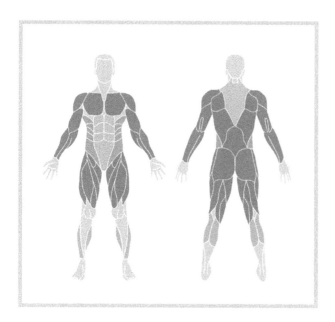

BULK ORDER

DAREBEE
WORKOUT
© darebee.com

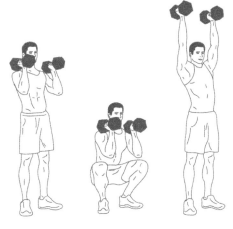

10 squat into shoulder press
5 sets in total
60 sec rest in between

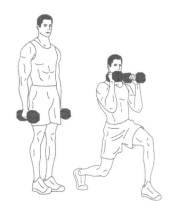

10 lunge into bicep curl
5 sets in total
60 sec rest in between

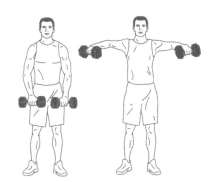

8 lateral raises
5 sets in total
60 sec rest in between

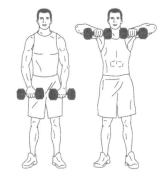

8 chest rows
5 sets in total
60 sec rest in between

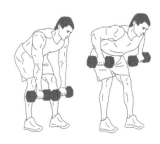

8 bent over rows
5 sets in total
60 sec rest in between

18 Butcher

The Butcher workout is designed to help you get stronger, denser and bigger muscles with a workout that uses weights to achieve the end result. Pick weights that will challenge you but do not be overly ambitious here. Each set piles on the pressure and as you go from one upper body muscle group to the next forcing the muscle adaptation response we need in order to make the body change.

Type: Classic
What It Works:

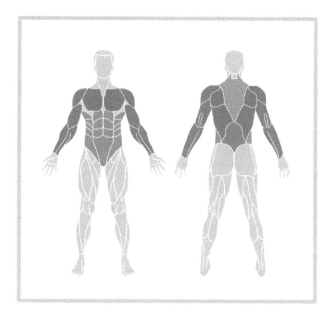

BUTCHER

DAREBEE WORKOUT © darebee.com

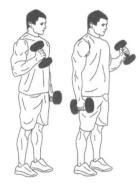

10 hammer curls
x **3 sets** in total
20 seconds rest
between sets

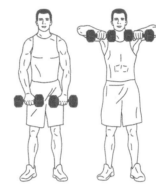

10 chest rows
x **3 sets** in total
20 seconds rest
between sets

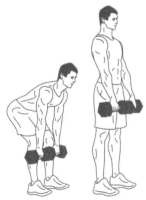

10 deadlifts
x **3 sets** in total
20 seconds rest
between sets

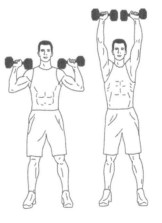

10 shoulder press
x **3 sets** in total
20 seconds rest
between sets

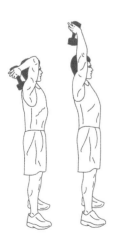

10 tricep extensions
x **3 sets** in total
20 seconds rest
between sets

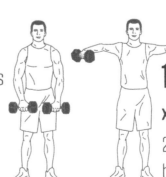

10 lateral raises
x **3 sets** in total
20 seconds rest
between sets

19 Catalyst

A catalyst is a tipping point. It makes a cascade of events possible and they lead to a transformation. The Catalyst workout then definitely lives up to its name. A series of equipment-based exercises help you begin the journey of transformation to a new level of strength and power.

Type: Classic
What It Works:

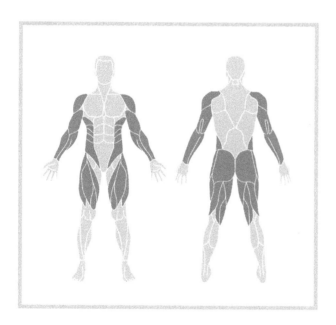

CATALYST

DAREBEE WORKOUT © darebee.com

2 minutes rest between exercises

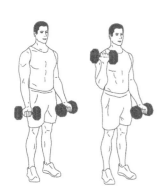

20 alt bicep curls
x 5 sets in total
20 seconds rest
between sets

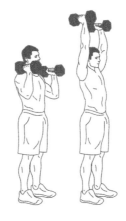

10 shoulder press
x 5 sets in total
20 seconds rest
between sets

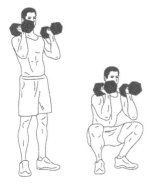

10 squats
x 5 sets in total
20 seconds rest
between sets

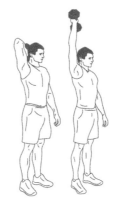

10 tricep extensions
x 5 sets in total
20 seconds rest
between sets

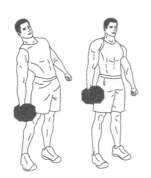

10 side tilts
x 5 sets in total
20 seconds rest
between sets

20 Chest & Back

If you have some dumbbells handy, you've got the recipe for a chest and back workout. The aptly named Chest & Back workout is an upperbody focused set of exercises that uses the number of reps to create a targeted training routine that works very specific muscle groups.

Type: Classic
What It Works:

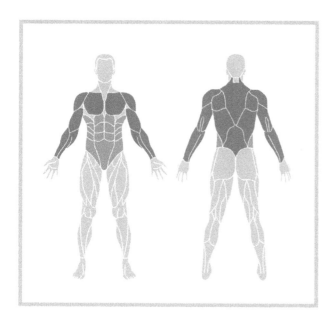

CHEST & BACK

DAREBEE WORKOUT
© darebee.com
60 seconds rest between exercises

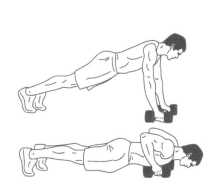

push-ups
12 / 10 / 8 / 6 reps
30 seconds rest between sets

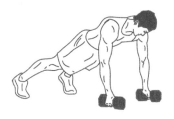
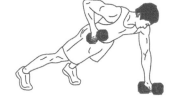

renegade rows
6 / 5 / 4 / 3 reps per arm
30 seconds rest between sets

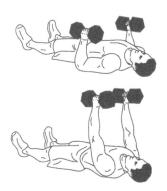

chest press
12 / 10 / 8 / 6 reps
30 seconds rest between sets

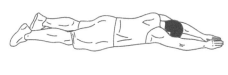
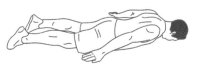

reverse angels
12 / 10 / 8 / 6 reps
30 seconds rest between sets

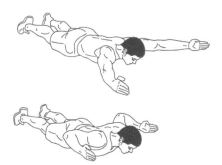

W-extensions
12 / 10 / 8 / 6 reps
30 seconds rest between sets

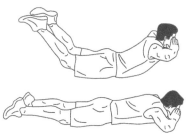

back extensions
12 / 10 / 8 / 6 reps
30 seconds rest between sets

21 Come Back Stronger

Come Back Stronger is a total body strength workout that uses dumbbells you have at your disposal to help you build strong muscles and powerful tendons. The results are increased, overall, muscle control. Greater power. More athleticism. A general sense of presence inside your body.

Type: Circuit
What It Works:

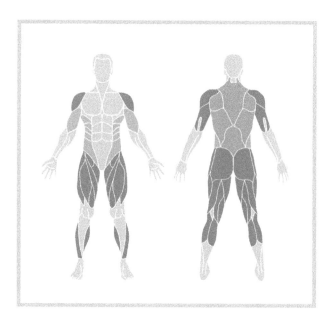

COME BACK
STRONGER

DAREBEE WORKOUT © darebee.com

LEVEL I 3 sets **LEVEL II** 5 sets **LEVEL III** 7 sets **REST** up to 2 minutes

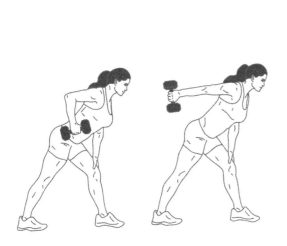

12 tricep extensions

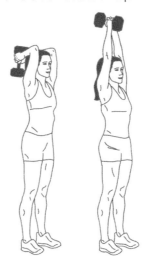

6 overhead tricep extensions

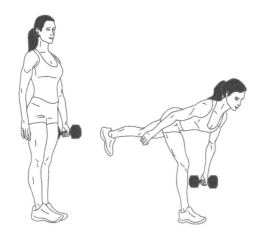

12 single leg deadlifts

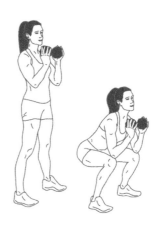

6 goblet squats

22   Cultivator

Cultivator is an upper body strength workout that helps activate the body's adaptive response and build stronger muscles. Included in your monthly set of workouts it will help not just your body's health but also your brain's.

Type: Circuit
What It Works:

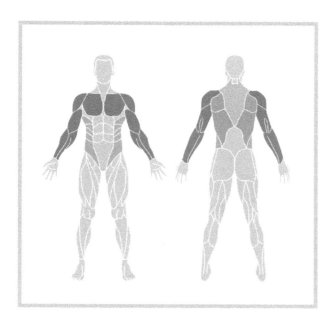

CULTIVATOR

DAREBEE WORKOUT © darebee.com

LEVEL I 3 sets **LEVEL II** 5 sets **LEVEL III** 7 sets **REST** up to 2 minutes

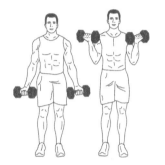

10 bicep curls

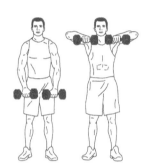

4 upright rows

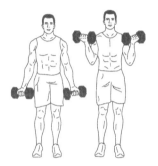

10 bicep curls

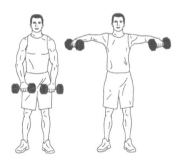

4 lateral raises

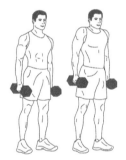

10 shrugs

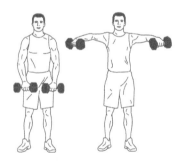

4 lateral raises

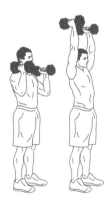

10 shoulder press

23 Digger

Digger lives up to its name. It tasks the entire body and you will definitely feel like you were digging, the day after. This is a strength training program that engages specific kinetic chains to generate the motion. The result is that muscles feel the load again and again. Great for activating the body's adaptive response which is what you want. It will definitely leave you feeling like you've done a strength workout.

Type: Circuit
What It Works:

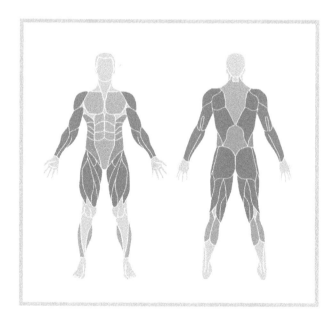

DIGGER

DAREBEE WORKOUT © darebee.com

LEVEL I 3 sets **LEVEL II** 5 sets **LEVEL III** 7 sets **REST** up to 2 minutes

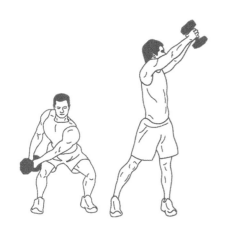

12 cross chops

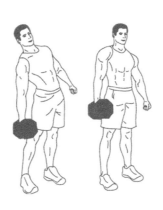

12 side bends

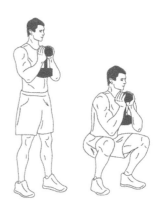

12 goblet squats

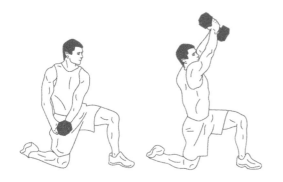

12 kneeling chops

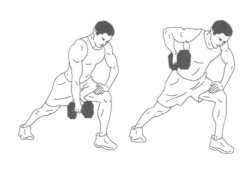

12 kneeling rows

24 Dumbbell Abs

Dumbbell Abs is a workout that proves you can't lift a weight with just your arms. Activating the body's kinetic chains requires a strong core and abs, especially if the power transfer is to be as lossless as possible. This is a workout that will put your abs and core to the test.

Type: Circuit
What It Works:

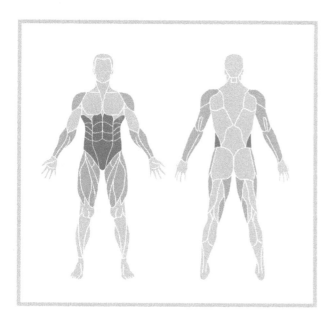

dumbbell abs

DAREBEE
WORKOUT
© darebee.com

LEVEL I	3 sets
LEVEL II	4 sets
LEVEL III	5 sets
REST	up to 2 minutes

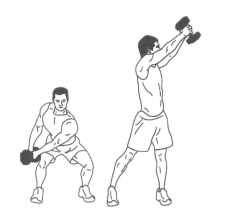

12 cross chops

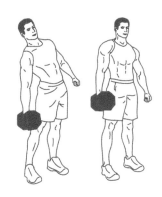

12 side bends

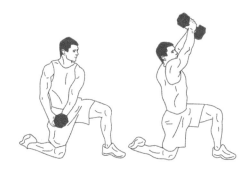

12 kneeling cross chops

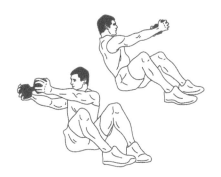

12 sitting twists

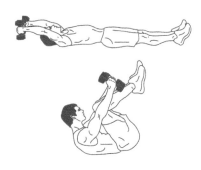

12 knee crunches

25 Dynamic Dumbbell

Nothing quite makes muscles and tendons work harder than the addition of a dumbbell to a workout. Dynamic Dumbbell lives up to its billing but there's a caveat in the workout. Listen to your body do not force the movements beyond your ability to control them and use a weight you can handle as opposed to one that will push you to your absolute limit.

Type: Circuit
What It Works:

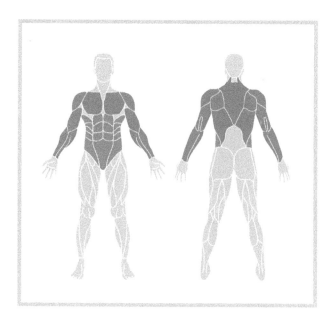

DYNAMIC DUMBBELL

DAREBEE WORKOUT
© darebee.com

LEVEL I 3 sets
LEVEL II 4 sets
LEVEL III 5 sets
REST 2 minutes

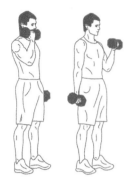

20 alt bicep curls

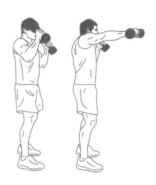

10 punches

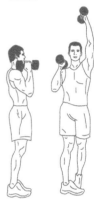

10 overhead punches

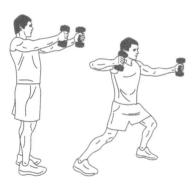

20 archers

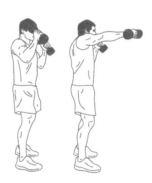

10 punches

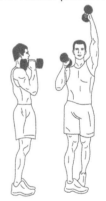

10 overhead punches

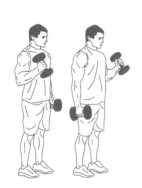

20 alt hammer curls

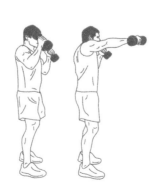

10 punches

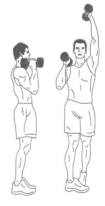

10 overhead punches

26   Endgame Plus

Full body workouts are great for days when you want to simply workout every muscle in your body but still want to be able to walk afterwards. Because the load applied is spread all over the intensity needle never goes into the red zone but that does not mean you're not going to sweat a lot while you're doing it. If anything, your body will definitely know it's being asked to delver the goods.

Type: Circuit
What It Works:

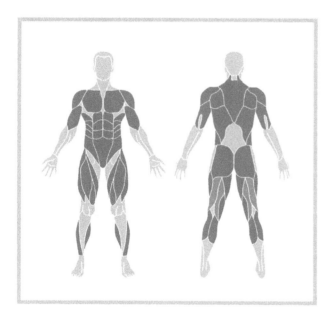

ENDGAME+

DAREBEE WORKOUT © darebee.com

LEVEL I 3 sets **LEVEL II** 5 sets **LEVEL III** 7 sets **REST** up to 2 minutes

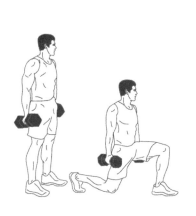

10 lunges

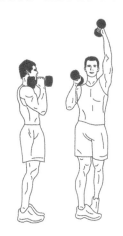

10 overhead punches

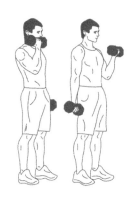

10 alt bicep curls

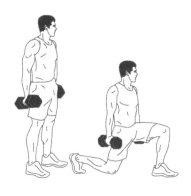

10 lunges

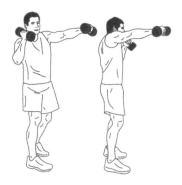

10 punches

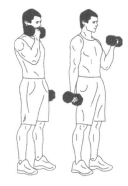

10 alt bicep curls

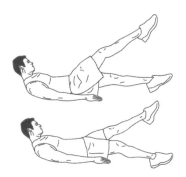

10 flutter kicks

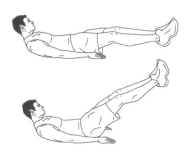

10 leg raises

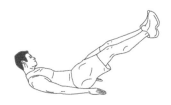

10-count raised leg hold

27 Enemy Lines Plus

The Enemy Lines+ workout focuses on upper body strength and speed without neglecting lower body strength. Upper body and core are focused upon, loading muscle groups in succession and shifting the load from one exercise to the next to allow some recovery to take place, on the fly. This is perfect for anyone doing boxing or martial arts and it will help increase upper body strength and power.

Type: Circuit
What It Works:

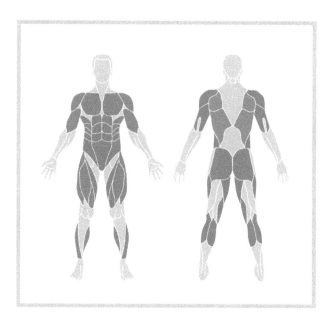

ENEMY LINES+

DAREBEE WORKOUT
© darebee.com
LEVEL I 3 sets
LEVEL II 5 sets
LEVEL III 7 sets
REST up to 2 minutes

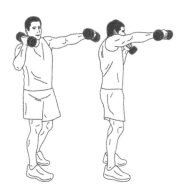

20 punches

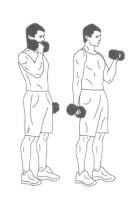

20 bicep curls

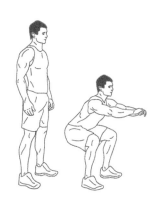

40 squats

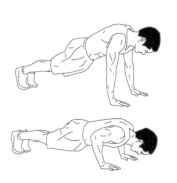

10 push-ups

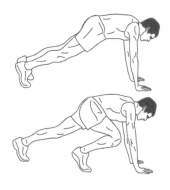

10 slow climbers

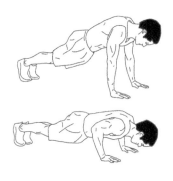

10 push-ups

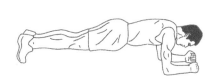

20-count plank

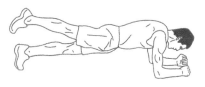

20-count plank

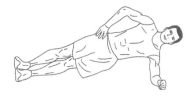

20-count plank

28　Epic Arms

Compound workouts combine exercise types to load the muscle group in a concentric and eccentric fashion, creating both a metabolic load (as the muscles increase their energy demand over time) and a cardiovascular one (with demand for oxygen rising and the need for metabolites to be removed increasing). Epic Arms works your arms (as expected) but also your core, abs and lower back as your body braces against the weights each time you curl and your torso twists every time you throw punches.

Type: Circuit
What It Works:

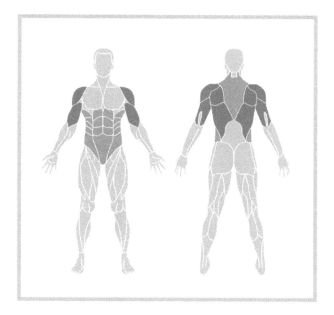

EPIC
ARMS

DAREBEE WORKOUT © darebee.com

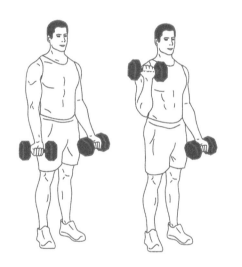

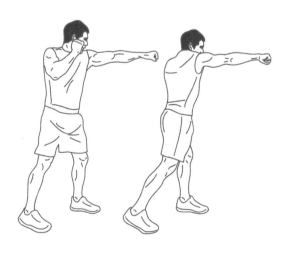

10 alt bicep curls

20 punches

10 alt bicep curls

20 punches

10 alt bicep curls

20 punches

10 alt bicep curls

20 punches

10 alt bicep curls

20 punches

done

29 Epic Gains

Muscles respond to stretching, tensing or fatigue and the Epic Gains workout combines all three in different ways to help your body feel stronger and be healthier. If you have a set of dumbbells this workout should be a go-to choice in your arsenal.

Type: Classic
What It Works:

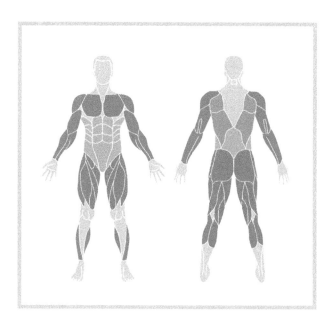

epic gains

DAREBEE WORKOUT © darebee.com

60 seconds rest
between exercises

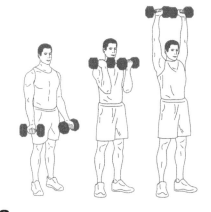

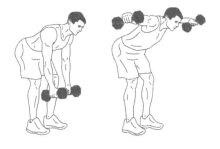

12 bicep curls into shoulder press
5 sets in total
60 sec rest in between

8 bent over lateral raises
5 sets in total
60 sec rest in between

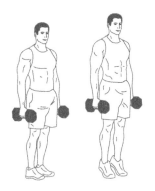

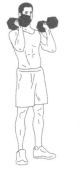

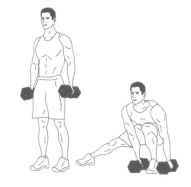

12 calf raises
5 sets in total
60 sec rest in between

12 squats
5 sets in total
60 sec rest in between

12 side lunges
5 sets in total
60 sec rest in between

30 Farmer

Farmer is a dumbbells-based workout that targets the entire body. It consistently loads specific muscle groups and recruits stabilizing tendons to create load points at specific muscle-to-bone angles. The result is that the body's adaptation response kicks in a lot faster. You will feel stronger, faster.

Type: Circuit
What It Works:

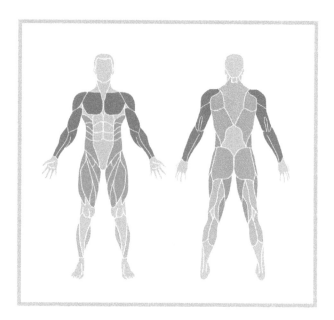

FARMER

DAREBEE WORKOUT © darebee.com

LEVEL I 3 sets **LEVEL II** 4 sets **LEVEL III** 5 sets **REST** up to 2 minutes

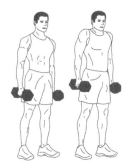

10 shrugs

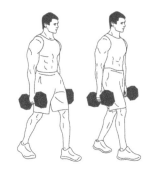

10 farmer carry steps

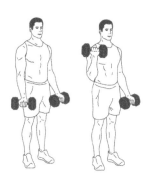

10 alt bicep curls

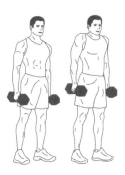

10 shrugs

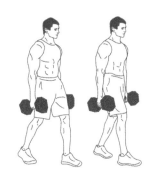

10 farmer carry steps

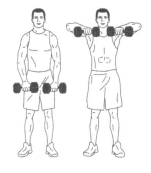

10 upright rows

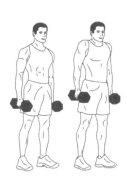

10 shrugs

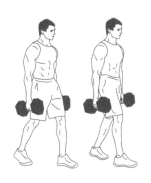

10 farmer carry steps

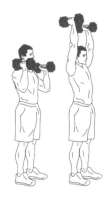

10 shoulder press

Full Body Built

Full Body Built is a dumbbell-based workout that targets virtually every large muscle group in the body to help you develop total body strength. Form is important in this workout and science shows that slowing down the speed of execution recruits more muscle fibers in each movement and delivers better results, faster.

Type: Classic
What It Works:

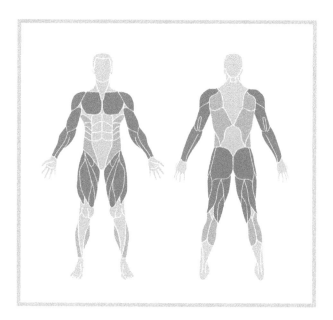

FULL BODY BUILT

12 reverse lunges **x 5 sets** in total
60 seconds rest between sets

12 squat into shoulder press **x 5 sets** in total
60 seconds rest between sets

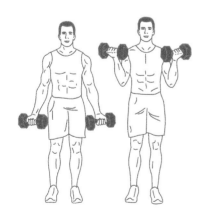

12 bicep curls **x 5 sets** in total
60 seconds rest between sets

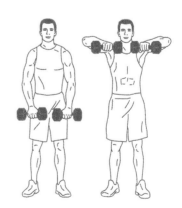

12 upright rows **x 5 sets** in total
60 seconds rest between sets

32   Fullbody Render Plus

FullBody Render is a Level IV full-body workout that also uses a set of weights to help you develop strength, balance, coordination and endurance.

Type: Circuit
What It Works:

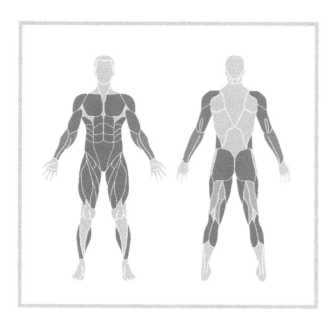

FULLBODY RENDER+

DAREBEE WORKOUT © darebee.com

LEVEL I 3 sets **LEVEL II** 5 sets **LEVEL III** 7 sets **REST** up to 2 minutes

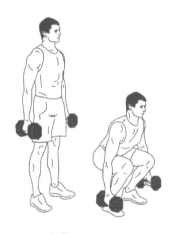

20 squats

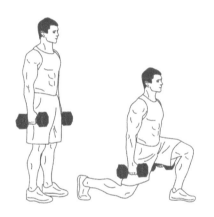

20 lunges

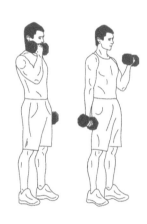

20 alt bicep curls

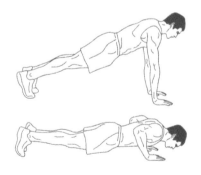

20 push-ups

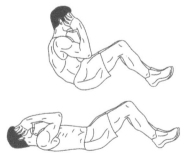

20 sit-ups

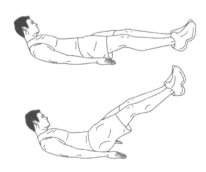

20 leg raises

33 Gainer

If you have some handy barbells and they are heavy enough to challenge you The Gainer workout will help you get strong all over. Designed to b a full body strength workout The Gainer uses a set of six exercises to load every muscle group, inducing fatigue and forcing the kind of change in the muscle fiber that results in strength gains.

Type: Classic
What It Works:

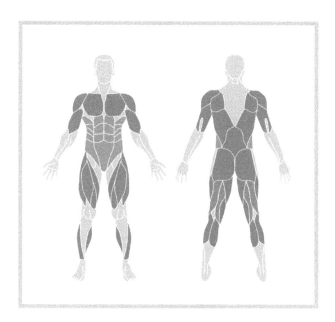

THE GAINER

DAREBEE WORKOUT © darebee.com

2 minutes rest between exercises

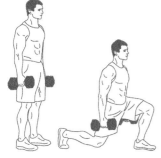

10 lunges
x 3 sets in total
20 seconds rest
between sets

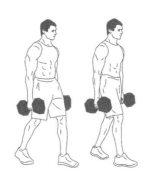

10steps farmer's walk
x 3 sets in total
20 seconds rest
between sets

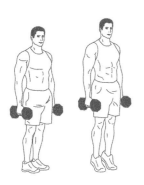

10 calf raises
x 3 sets in total
20 seconds rest
between sets

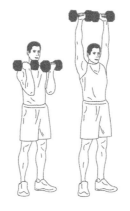

10 Arnold's press
x 3 sets in total
20 seconds rest
between sets

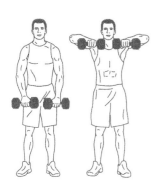

10 upright rows
x 3 sets in total
20 seconds rest
between sets

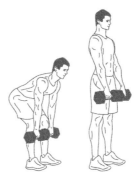

10 deadlifts
x 3 sets in total
20 seconds rest
between sets

Glutes Sculpt

Although we don't really get to think about them because they are well, behind us glutes are key to generating power when we need it the most. They affect our posture, enhance our jumping and kicking, power our running and sprinting and amplify pretty much every move we make. Glutes Sculpt will help you turn them into a true powerhouse. Grab some weights and get to work!

Type: Classic
What It Works:

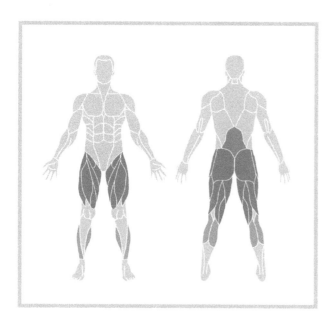

GLUTES

WORKOUT BY © darebee.com

SCULPT

2 minutes rest between exercises

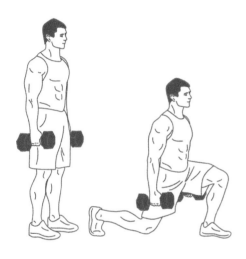

forward lunges
12, 10, 8, 6 (both legs)
30 seconds rest

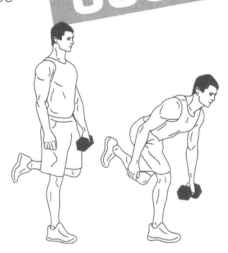

single leg deadlifts
12, 10, 8, 6 (both legs)
30 seconds rest

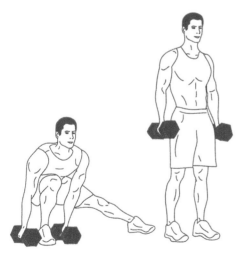

deep side lunges
12, 10, 8, 6 (both legs)
30 seconds rest

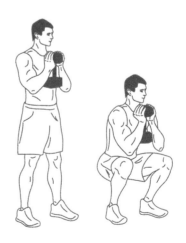

goblet squats
10, 8, 6, 4
30 seconds rest

35 Goliath

If you have a pair of dumbbells lying around then the Goliath workout will help you put them to good use. That will be good for them, of course, plus it will be great for you as you will get a decent workout.

Type: Classic
What It Works:

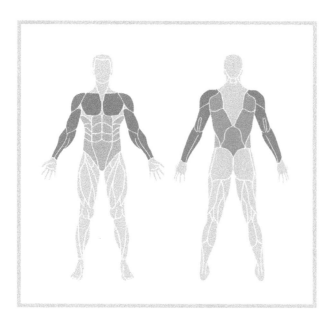

GOLIATH

DAREBEE WORKOUT © darebee.com

2 minutes rest between exercises

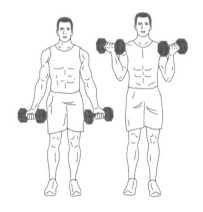

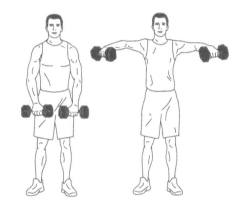

12 biceps curls **x 5 sets** in total
60 seconds rest between sets

6 lateral raises **x 5 sets** in total
60 seconds rest between sets

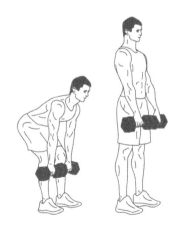

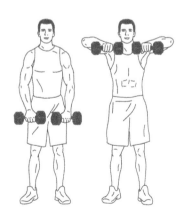

6 deadlifts **x 5 sets** in total
60 seconds rest between sets

6 upright rows **x 5 sets** in total
60 seconds rest between sets

36 Hammer

If you have some dumbbells lying around (or can get hold of some makeshift weights) you can use your body to train with the load of an imaginary weapon (hammer, sword, axe or pike). When loaded during ballistic exercises muscles perform differently, calling on many supporting muscle groups to help maintain the body's balance so this can be quite the challenge.

Type: Circuit
What It Works:

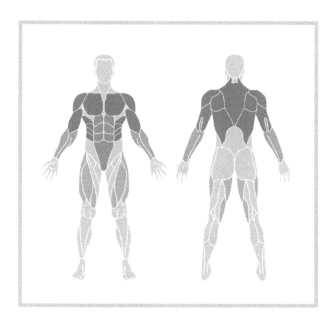

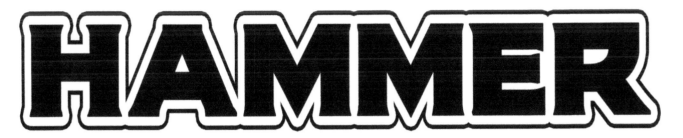

HAMMER

DAREBEE WORKOUT © darebee.com

3 sets | 60 seconds rest between sets

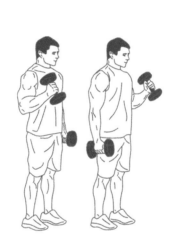

10 hammer curls

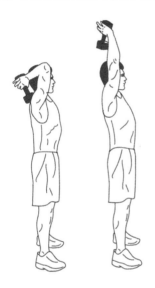

10 tricep extensions

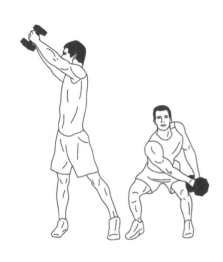

10 cross chops

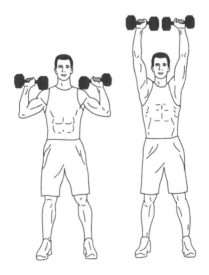

6 shoulder press

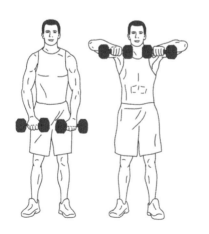

6 upright rows

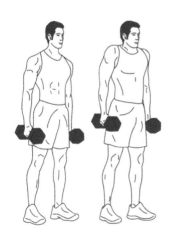

6 shrugs

37 Hardgainer

The Hardgainer is a complete upper body (arms + back) workout designed to primarily add size. The rep count is low so go for heavier weight. If you don't have dumbbells that are 16lb+ (8kg+) on hand, use smaller weights but do each rep as slowly as possible.

Type: Classic
What It Works:

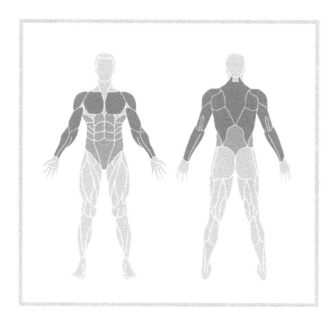

HARDGAINER

DAREBEE WORKOUT © darebee.com

2 minutes rest between exercises

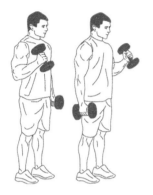

hammer curls
12, 10, 8, 6 reps
20 seconds rest
between sets

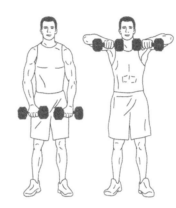

upward rows
12, 10, 8, 6 reps
20 seconds rest
between sets

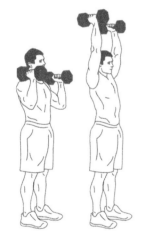

shoulder press
12, 10, 8, 6 reps
20 seconds rest
between sets

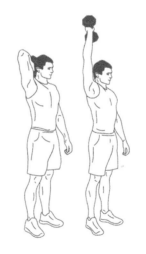

tricep extensions
6, 5, 4, 3 reps each
20 seconds rest
between sets

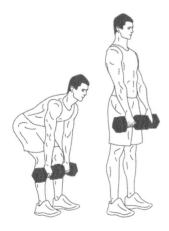

deadlifts
12, 10, 8, 6 reps
20 seconds rest
between sets

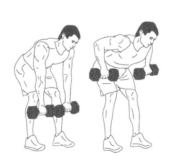

bent over rows
12, 10, 8, 6 reps
20 seconds rest
between sets

38   HD Arms

If you have a pair of light dumbbells, two arms and a bathroom you're in for a transformative exercise regime. The reason you need dumbbells is self-explanatory and the same should be said for the pair of arms but the bathroom needs a little more explanation. It's probably the easiest place to place a couple of dumbbells and go through the exercise routine every time you find yourself there. Smart training is all about lowering the threshold barriers by getting rid of the perceived obstacles to exercise. This is a routine you'll love and it will change you.

Type: Circuit
What It Works:

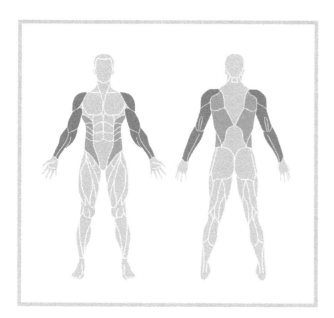

HD ARMS

DAREBEE WORKOUT © darebee.com

Use light 4kg (9lb) dumbbells and <u>go to failure each time</u>
Repeat the workout 4-5 times during the day, whenever you can
Increase the reps the moment you feel you can do more.

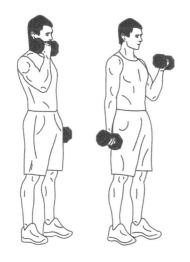

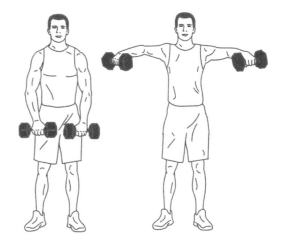

alternating dumbbell curls

lateral raises

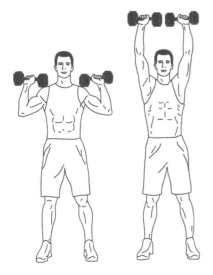

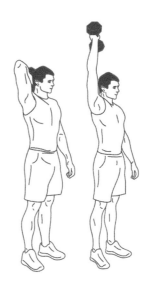

shoulder press

tricep extensions

39 Heavy Duty

Heavy Duty is a workout for anyone who has a couple of 5kg+ (10lb+) dumbbells lying around as a minimum weight and is ready to do some heavy duty work (pun entirely intended). This is a strength workout and stronger muscles allow you to do everything more easily.

Type: Circuit
What It Works:

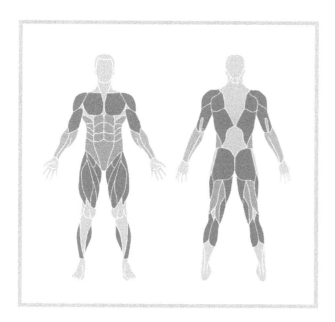

HEAVY DUTY

WORKOUT BY DAREBEE
© darebee.com
5 sets in total
2 min rest between sets

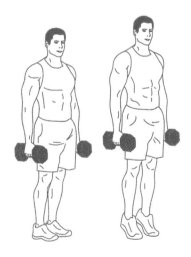

20combos squat + shoulder press   **20combos** lunge + hammer curl

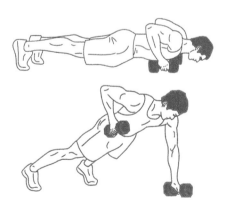

20 calf raises   **20** renegade row push-ups

40 Hephaestus

If you're working the forge you need the bulk. So the Hephaestus workout gets you using your weights for some resistance work that'll help your muscles, add density to your bones and help your brain stay healthy as you age. Resistance training should always be part of your general fitness routine.

Type: Classic
What It Works:

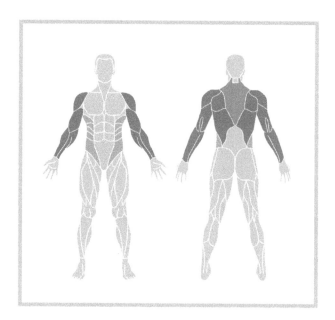

HEPHAESTUS

DAREBEE WORKOUT © darebee.com

2 minutes rest between exercises

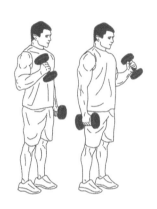

12 hammer curls
x 5 sets in total
20 seconds rest
between sets

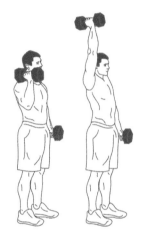

12 shoulder press
x 5 sets in total
20 seconds rest
between sets

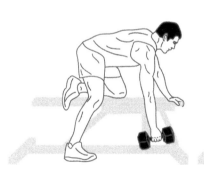

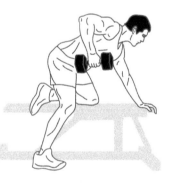

12 rows
x 5 sets in total
20 seconds rest
between sets

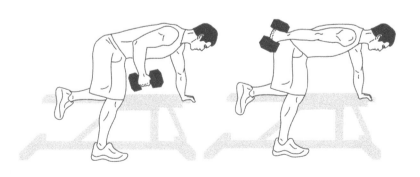

12 tricep extensions
x 5 sets in total
20 seconds rest
between sets

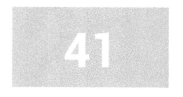 # Home Upperbody Tone

The upper body takes a lot of work and, because of our modern lifestyle, never quite gets enough. The Home Upperbody Tone workout redresses that imbalance a little by providing you with a dumbbell workout that will engage all the major muscle groups and help your body get stronger, look more toned and feel better.

Type: Circuit
What It Works:

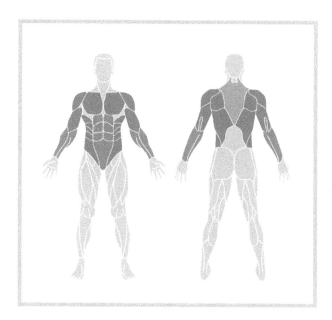

HOME UPPERBODY TONE

DAREBEE WORKOUT
© darebee.com
Level I 3 sets
Level II 4 sets
Level III 5 sets
2 minutes rest

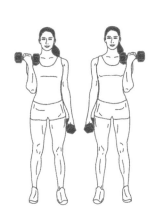

20 alternating bicep curls

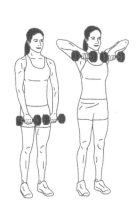

10 upright rows

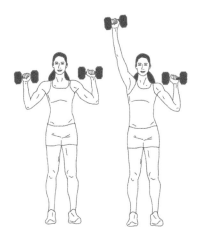

10 alternating shoulder press

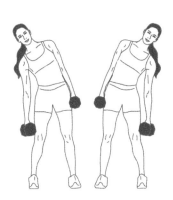

10 side bends

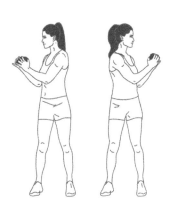

10 core twists

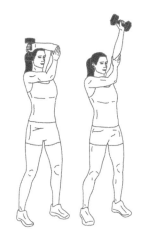

20 tricep extensions

42. Hunter Plus

If you had to hunt for your food you'd push yourself past every limit and overcome every barrier to catch your next meal. Hunter is a workout that will make your muscles work hard. It's not very heavy on aerobics but it does demand a lot from your muscles. Perform each exercise slowly, focusing on form and perfect execution. Keep your punches at chin height at all times, your push up deep, your body straight and your squats really deep. Suggested dumbbell weight: 2-3 kg (5-7lb) max.

Type: Circuit
What It Works:

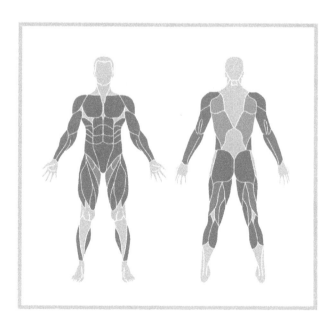

HUNTER+

DAREBEE WORKOUT © darebee.com

LEVEL I 3 sets **LEVEL II** 5 sets **LEVEL III** 7 sets **REST** up to 2 minutes

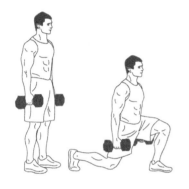

10 lunges

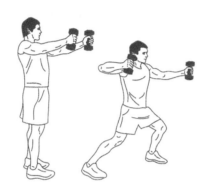

20 archer lunges

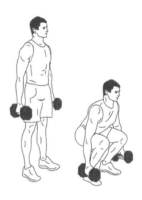

20 squats

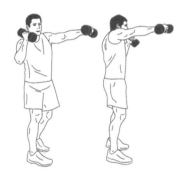

20 punches

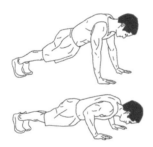

10 push-ups

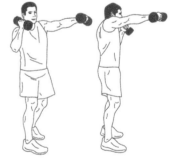

20 punches

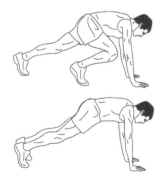

10 climbers

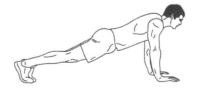

20-count plank

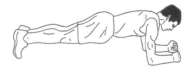

20-count elbow plank

Hybrid

Despite the strength we can generate, our upper body is relatively weak for our size in the animal kingdom. We can address some of this imbalance with The Hybrid workout, specifically designed to mix bodyweight exercises and dumbbells using both concentric and eccentric muscle movements. The result is an upper body strength workout that will help you get stronger and increase your body's resistance to fatigue.

Type: Circuit
What It Works:

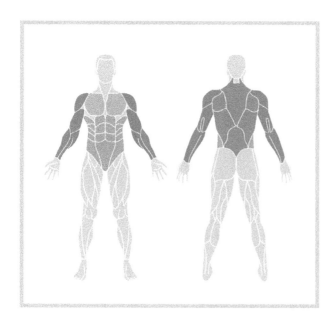

THE HYBRID

DAREBEE WORKOUT © darebee.com

LEVEL I 3 sets **LEVEL II** 5 sets **LEVEL III** 7 sets **REST** up to 2 minutes

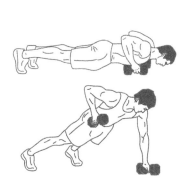

10 push-up renegade rows

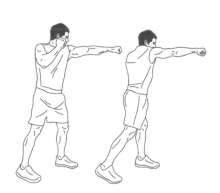

20 punches

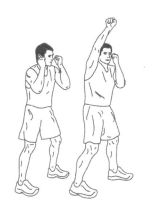

20 overhead punches

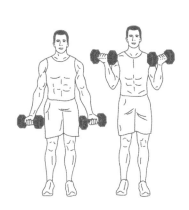

10 bicep curls

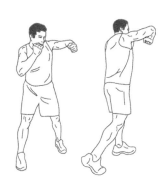

20 hooks

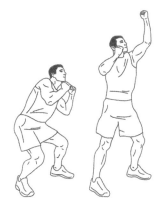

20 uppercuts

44   Iron Dragon

Resistance training strengthens individual muscle fibers, leads to stronger muscles and stronger bones. Stronger bones play a role in cognitive health. The Iron Dragon workout helps you get stronger inside and out. All you need is a set of dumbbells and the time to lift them. The rest gets taken care of for you.

Type: Classic
What It Works:

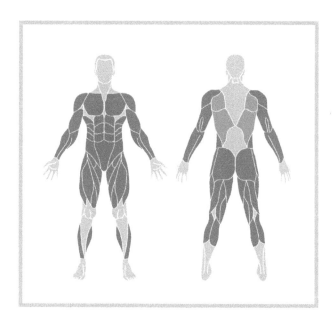

IRON DRAGON

DAREBEE WORKOUT © darebee.com

2 minutes rest between exercises

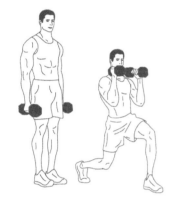

12 lunge hammer curls
x 4 sets in total
20 seconds rest
between sets

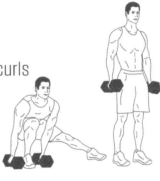

12 side lunges
x 4 sets in total
20 seconds rest
between sets

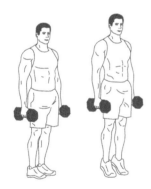

8 calf raises
x 4 sets in total
20 seconds rest
between sets

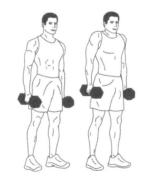

6 shrugs
x 4 sets in total
20 seconds rest
between sets

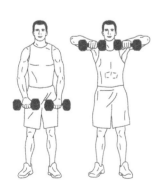

8 chest rows
x 4 sets in total
20 seconds rest
between sets

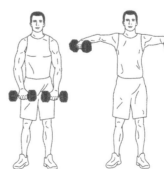

6 lateral raises
x 4 sets in total
20 seconds rest
between sets

45 Ironheart

If you have a couple of dumbbells handy you can feel the benefits of the Ironheart, full body, muscle-toning workout. Its series of dynamic exercises with the added weight trigger the body's adaptive response and help you become stronger, faster.

Type: Circuit
What It Works:

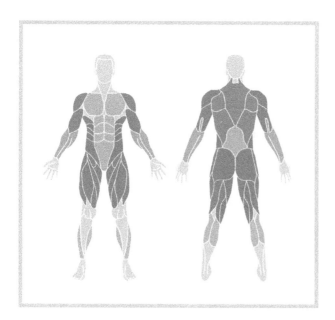

IRONHEART

DAREBEE WORKOUT © darebee.com

LEVEL I 3 sets **LEVEL II** 5 sets **LEVEL III** 7 sets **REST** up to 2 minutes

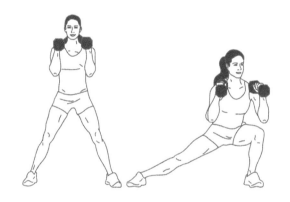

12 side lunges

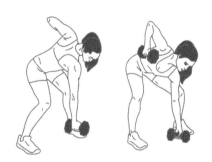

12 alternating bent over rows

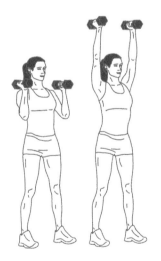

6 shoulder press

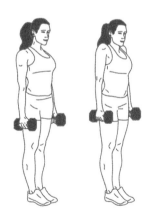

6 shrugs

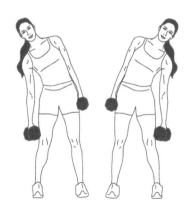

12 side bends

46 Iron Will

Iron Will is a dumbbells-based workout that will help your body develop strength, stability, coordination and power through a series of resistance exercises. The activation of the body's back and front kinetic chains and its core delivers performance benefits way above the difficulty level of this workout. This is one to keep in mind for the days when you want to reach for those dumbbells you have lying around.

Type: Circuit
What It Works:

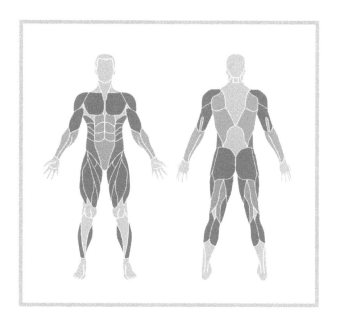

IRON WILL

DAREBEE WORKOUT
© darebee.com
LEVEL I 3 sets
LEVEL II 4 sets
LEVEL III 5 sets
REST up to 2 minutes

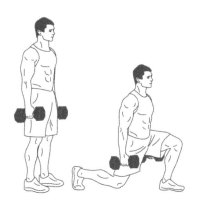

10 lunges

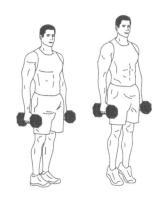

10 calf raises

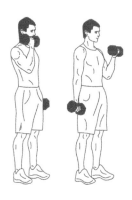

10 alt bicep curls

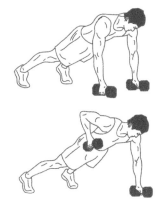

10 renegade rows

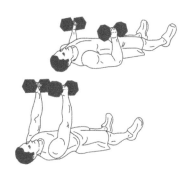

10 chest press

Jacked

If you have a couple of dumbbells handy and are ready to apply an extrinsic load to the body then get ready for a workout that will leave you feeling Jacked for the day and a little sore the day after. This is a full body workout and to get the most out of it you'll need to get your breathing right and establish a rhythm that works for you. That actually will make a huge difference to how much you burn in this particular workout as well as how you feel afterwards.

Type: Classic
What It Works:

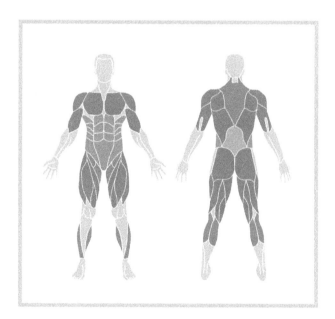

JACKED

DAREBEE WORKOUT © darebee.com

2 minutes rest between exercises

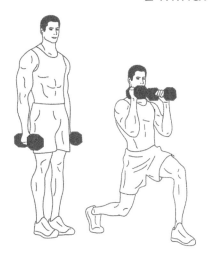

lunge + bicep curls
12, 10, 8, 6 reps
20 seconds rest between sets

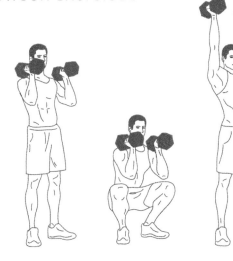

squat + shoulder press
12, 10, 8, 6 reps
20 seconds rest between sets

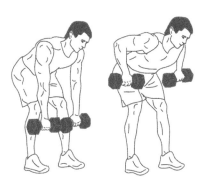

bent over rows
12, 10, 8, 6 reps
20 seconds rest between sets

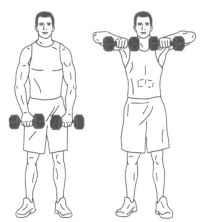

upright rows
12, 10, 8, 6 reps
20 seconds rest between sets

48 Jungle

A total body workout that builds serious muscle strength and still works your cardiovascular and aerobic systems can only be called Welcome To The Jungle. This is a workout that activates the body's kinetic chains to help muscles get stronger and your body hardened to fatigue.

Type: Circuit
What It Works:

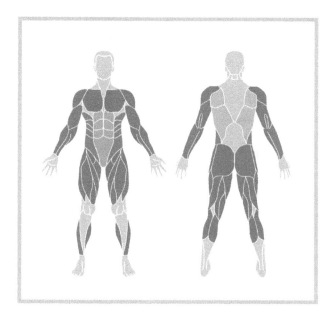

WELCOME TO THE
JUNGLE

DAREBEE WORKOUT © darebee.com
30 seconds rest between sets

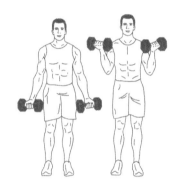

SET 1
20 bicep curls
2 push-ups
20 high knees

SET 2
18 bicep curls
3 push-ups
18 high knees

SET 3
16 bicep curls
4 push-ups
16 high knees

SET 4
14 bicep curls
5 push-ups
14 high knees

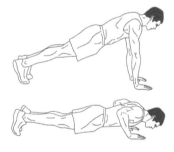

SET 5
12 bicep curls
6 push-ups
12 high knees

SET 6
10 bicep curls
7 push-ups
10 high knees

SET 7
8 bicep curls
8 push-ups
8 high knees

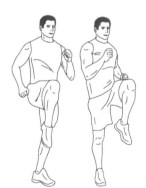

49   Lift & Tone

Combining weights with callisthenics Lift & Tone is a workout that delivers quite the kick despite the fact that each set is relatively short. This means that it targets the whole body and recruits a lot of satellite muscle groups while it does it. So, you really need to have this on your horizon regardless.

Type: Classic
What It Works:

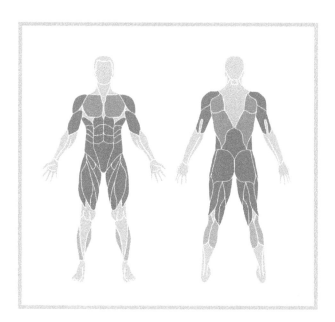

lift &
tone

DAREBEE WORKOUT © darebee.com

2 minutes rest between exercises

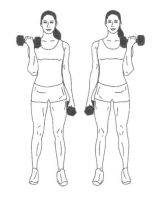

20 alt bicep curls
x 4 sets in total
20 seconds rest
between sets

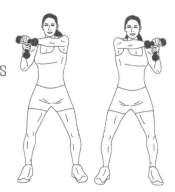

20 punches
x 4 sets in total
20 seconds rest
between sets

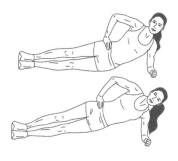

20 side bridges
x 4 sets in total
20 seconds rest
between sets

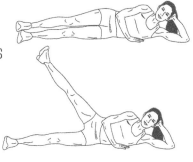

20 side leg raises
x 4 sets in total
20 seconds rest
between sets

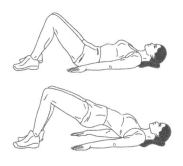

20 bridges
x 4 sets in total
20 seconds rest
between sets

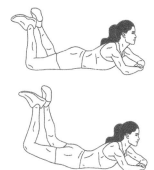

20 glute flex
x 4 sets in total
20 seconds rest
between sets

50 Like A Boss

If you own a set of dumbbells the Like A Boss workout will help you take your fitness up a notch or two through a set of exercises that activate the upper body. This workout will help you develop strength and core stability as well as challenge your body's ability to get blood quickly to large muscles.

Type: Circuit
What It Works:

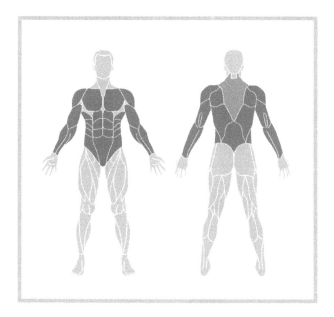

LIKE A BOSS

LEVEL I 3 sets **LEVEL II** 4 sets **LEVEL III** 5 sets **REST** up to 2 minutes

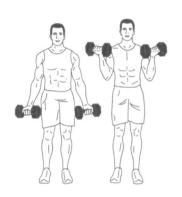

16 bicep curls

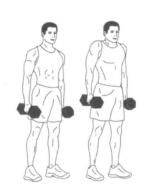

8 shrugs

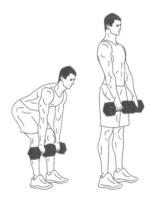

8 deadlifts

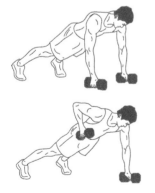

16 renegade rows

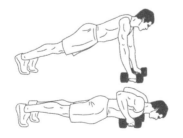

to fatigue push-ups

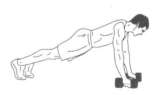

8-count plank hold

51 Mammoth

The Mammoth is a dumbbells workout designed to help build or maintain muscle. Its emphasis on strength helps maintain good strong bones which, in turn, aid in maintaining brain health. Because there is no real separation of the body and brain what makes one strong, also strengthens the other.

Type: Classic
What It Works:

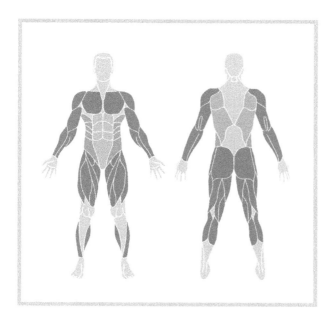

THE MAMMOTH

DAREBEE WORKOUT © darebee.com

2 minutes rest between exercises

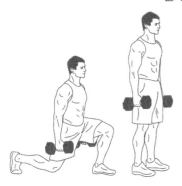

16 reverse lunges
x 5 sets in total
30 seconds rest
between sets

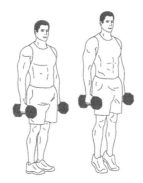

16 calf raises
x 5 sets in total
30 seconds rest
between sets

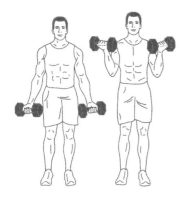

12 bicep curls
x 5 sets in total
30 seconds rest
between sets

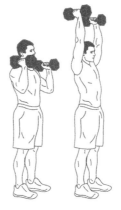

12 shoulder press
x 5 sets in total
30 seconds rest
between sets

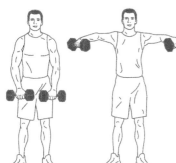

8 lateral raises
x 5 sets in total
30 seconds rest
between sets

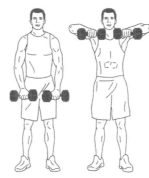

8 upright rows
x 5 sets in total
30 seconds rest
between sets

52   Mason Plus

Increase the resistance bodyweight training adds to your workout by picking up a pair of barbels and stepping up onto a box or any other convenient, stable base. The Mason workout is a fully cardiovascular activity, performed with precision of movement and attention to technique so that it does not turn into an aerobic exercise, it will take each major muscle group through its full range of movement. If you're looking for increased body strength then this will definitely help you out. Try and use barbels that will challenge your upper body strength.

Type: Circuit
What It Works:

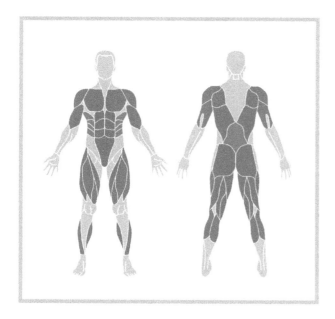

MASON+

DAREBEE WORKOUT © darebee.com

10 sets or as many as you can do | up to 2 minutes rest between sets

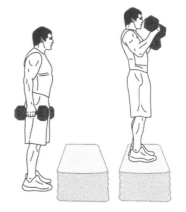

10 bicep curl steps

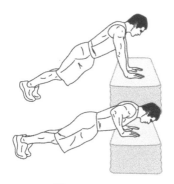

5 push-ups

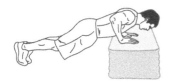

10-count push-up hold

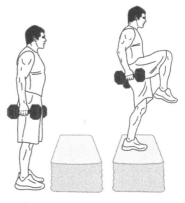

10 dumbbell step-ups

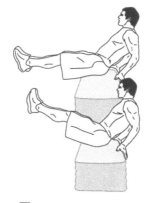

5 leg raises

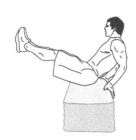

10-count raised leg hold

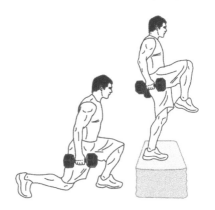

10 dumbbell step-up reverse lunges

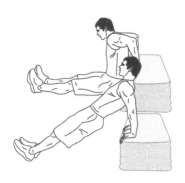

5 tricep dips

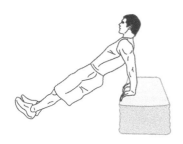

10-count tricep dip hold

53 Mave

The Mave workout will force you to work your upper body, activating the adaptive response and helping you become stronger. It will also give you greater control of your muscles and help improve bone density which contributes to your cognitive health.

Type: Circuit
What It Works:

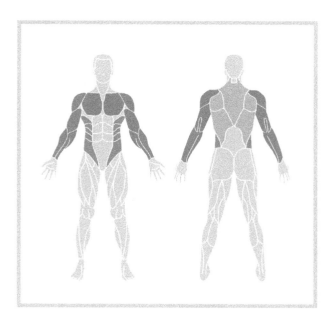

MAVE

DAREBEE WORKOUT © darebee.com

LEVEL I 3 sets **LEVEL II** 5 sets **LEVEL III** 7 sets **REST** up to 2 minutes

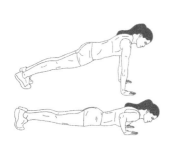

4 push-ups

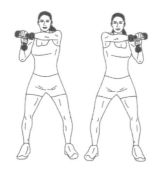

20 punches

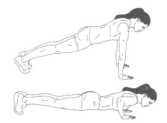

4 push-ups

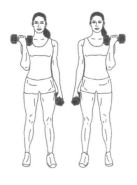

20 alt bicep curls

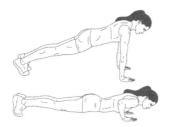

4 push-ups

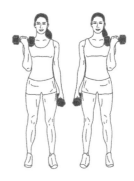

20 alt bicep curls

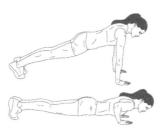

4 push-ups

54   Meta Burn

Meta Burn is a workout that targets the upper body muscles to deliver a sense of constant load as you go from one exercise to the other. If you have a pair of dumbbells lying around then this is the perfect workout to put them to good use.

Type: Circuit
What It Works:

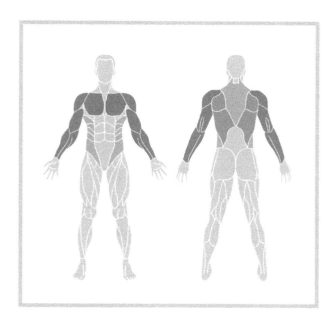

META BURN

DAREBEE WORKOUT © darebee.com

LEVEL I 3 sets **LEVEL II** 5 sets **LEVEL III** 7 sets **REST** 20 seconds

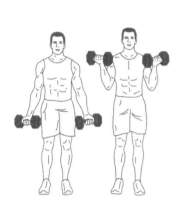

6 bicep curls

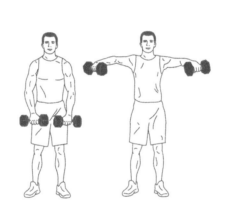

6 lateral raises

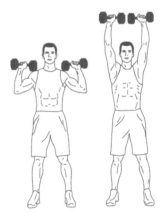

6 shoulder press

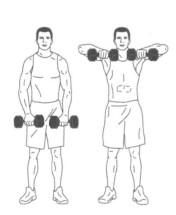

6 upright rows

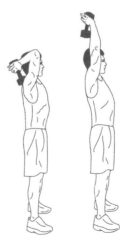

6 tricep extensions

55 Moving Mountains

Take two dumbbells, add one warm body, mix in some focus, sprinkle attention to form liberally, stir for five sets. Don't forget to break between each set. The recipe for success is in the Moving Mountains workout. Designed to specifically target all the major muscle groups in the body it will leave you feeling stronger than before.

Type: Circuit
What It Works:

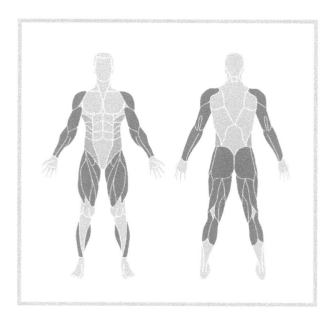

MOVING MOUNTAINS

DAREBEE WORKOUT © darebee.com

5 sets   2 minutes rest between sets

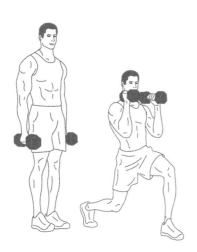

10 lunge hammer curls

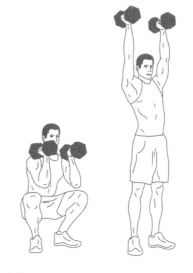

10 squat shoulder press

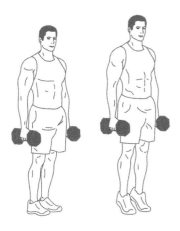

10 calf raises

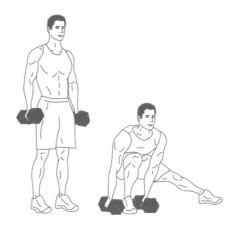

10 deep side lunges

56

Muscle Factory Lowerbody

The lower body is a paradox. Handling the whole body's weight it only gets better if it is put under a load greater than what it would normally be expected to carry. If you have some dumbbells lying around this is the perfect opportunity to make your body feel lighter. Work through the exercises and reap the benefits.

Type: Classic
What It Works:

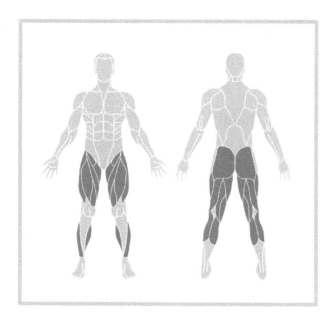

MUSCLE
FACTORY
DAREBEE WORKOUT © darebee.com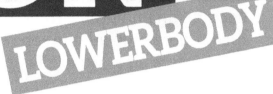

2 minutes rest between exercises

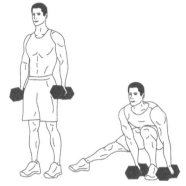

8 side lunges
x 5 sets in total
30 seconds rest
between sets

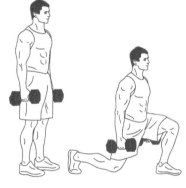

8 lunges
x 5 sets in total
30 seconds rest
between sets

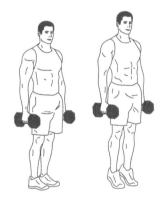

8 calf raises
x 5 sets in total
30 seconds rest
between sets

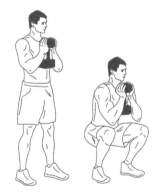

8 goblet squats
x 5 sets in total
30 seconds rest
between sets

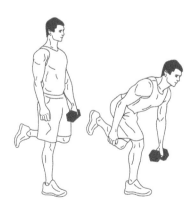

8 single leg deadlifts
x 5 sets in total
30 seconds rest
between sets

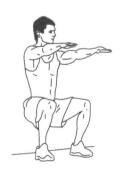

2 minutes
wall-sit

57

Muscle Factory Upperbody

Weights deliver an extraneous load to the body which means that they become an immutable force that doesn't lessen as the muscles fatigue. It then triggers the adaptation response which leads to increase in strength and muscle size. Muscle Factory is a workout that cleverly uses this principle to challenge a number of upper body muscle groups. Use your breathing when lifting to tighten your abs and also engage your core a little more and you've got yourself the kind of workout you feel you've done the day after.

Type: Classic
What It Works:

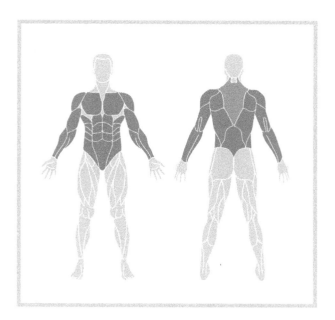

MUSCLE FACTORY

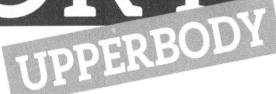

DAREBEE WORKOUT © **darebee.com**

2 minutes rest between exercises

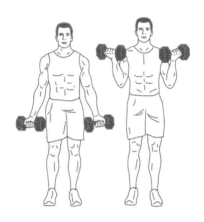

10 bicep curls
x 5 sets in total
30 seconds rest
between sets

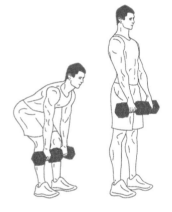

10 deadlifts
x 5 sets in total
30 seconds rest
between sets

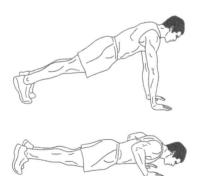

20 push-ups
x 5 sets in total
30 seconds rest
between sets

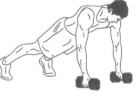
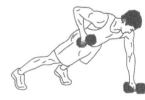

10 renegade rows
x 5 sets in total
30 seconds rest
between sets

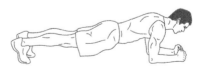
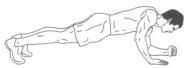
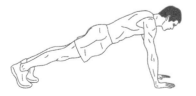

10 up and down planks **x 5 sets** in total | 30 seconds rest between sets

58 Ox

Unleash your inner work beast. Grab some dumbbells and work your upper body to activate the cellular adaptive response that will give you a stronger self. Ox is a workout designed to help you build a stronger upper body.

Type: Circuit
What It Works:

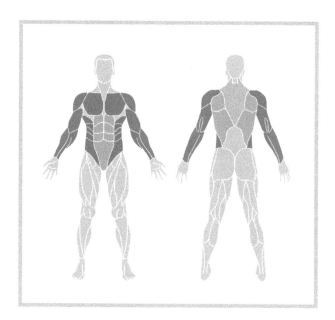

OX

DAREBEE WORKOUT
© darebee.com

Level I 3 sets
Level II 5 sets
Level III 7 sets
2 minutes rest

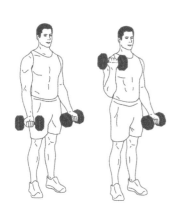

20 alt bicep curls

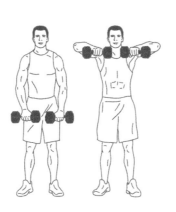

10 upright rows

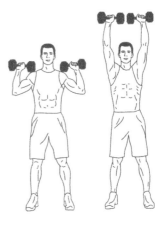

10 shoulder press

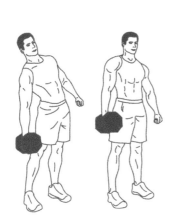

20 side bends

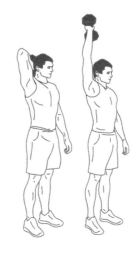

20 tricep extensions

59 Pixie

The moment you add weights and some core/balance exercises together you have an upper body workout that will work not just muscles but also tendons and core and help you improve your balance and stability. The Pixie workout does all of that, exactly. It will also challenge your cardiovascular system as the body pumps blood to all the upper body large, muscle groups.

Type: Circuit
What It Works:

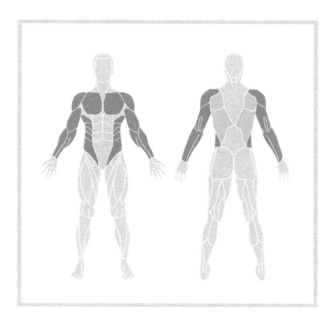

pixie

DAREBEE WORKOUT © darebee.com

LEVEL I 3 sets **LEVEL II** 4 sets **LEVEL III** 5 sets **REST** up to 2 minutes

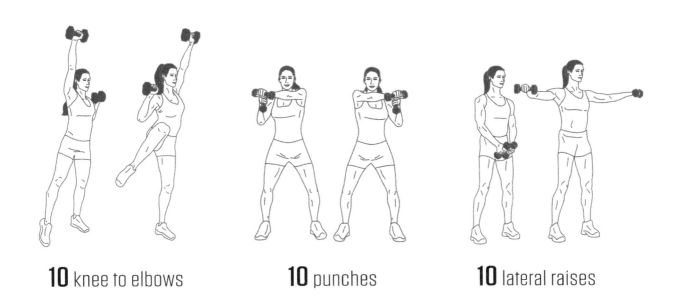

10 knee to elbows   **10** punches   **10** lateral raises

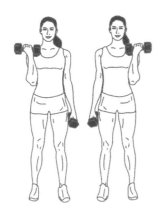   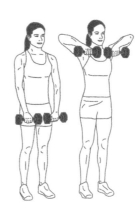

10 bicep curls   **10** chest rows

60 Power 10

Level up your arms' power level with a little help from your common household furniture, some dumbbells (we provide alternatives if you don't have these handy) and a little perseverance. The results will be toned, stronger arms that will let you do everything much easier and way better and that includes gaming. This is very much an intensive transformational exercise that will increase your upper body strength.

Type: Circuit
What It Works:

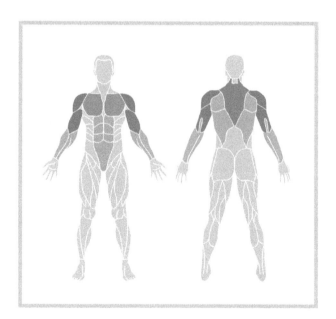

Power 10

DAREBEE WORKOUT © darebee.com

3 sets | 60 seconds rest between sets

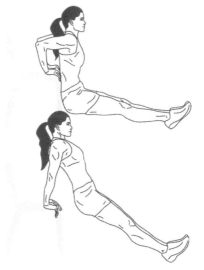

20 tricep dips

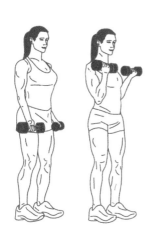

20 bicep curls

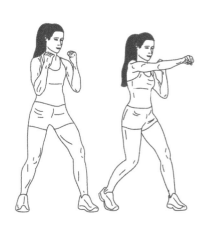

20 punches

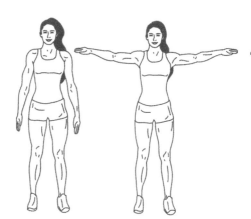

20 arm raises

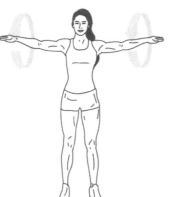

20 raised arm circles

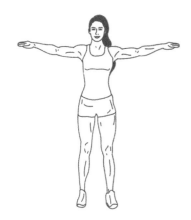

20sec raised arm hold

TIPS Don't have dumbbells? Use water battles or cans of beans instead.
Keep your arms up between raised arm circles and raised arm hold.

Power 18

The path to power level 9000 starts with a single lift. By working within your comfort levels here you begin the journey that will take you outside them. So, pick up a pair of your favourite dumbbells and begin the journey to the outer levels of your capabilities.

Type: Classic
What It Works:

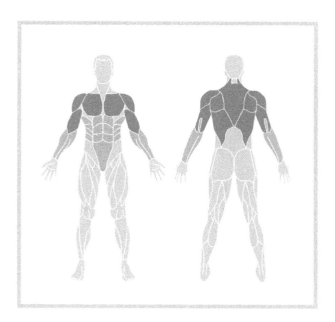

Power 18

DAREBEE WORKOUT © darebee.com
Use comfortable weights for this routine.
Pick up heavier weights the moment it gets easier.

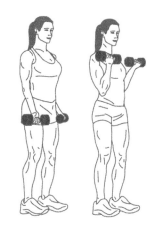

10 alt bicep curls
3 sets | 20 sec rest

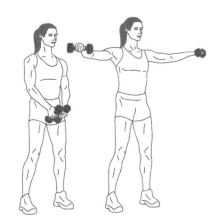

5 lateral raises
3 sets | 20 sec rest

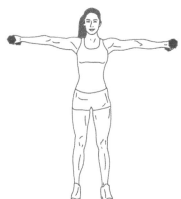

10-count hold
once

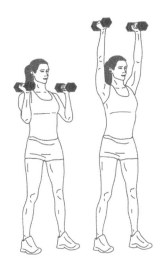

5 shoulder presses
3 sets | 20 sec rest

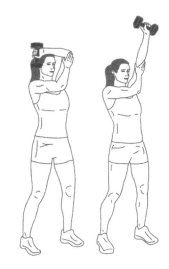

10 tricep extensions
3 sets | 20 sec rest

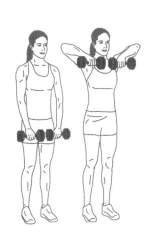

10 upright rows
3 sets | 20 sec rest

62   Power 20

Our arms are our primary weapon, toolset and creative implement all
rolled into one. Strong, capable arms unleash our own abilities, give us the
confidence to do the things we want to do and allow us to feel great inside
our bodies. The Power 20 workout is all about levelling up. Acquiring more
strength, more muscle endurance, more capability which means you will be
able to do more with it. Don't settle for playing the 'game' at the same level
all the time. Challenge yourself and open up fresh achievements to unlock.

Type: Classic
What It Works:

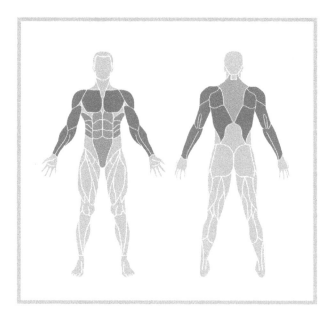

Power 20

DAREBEE WORKOUT © darebee.com
Use weights you can just do this routine with.
Pick up heavier weights the moment it gets easier.

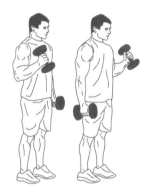

10 alt hammer curls
3 sets | 20 sec rest

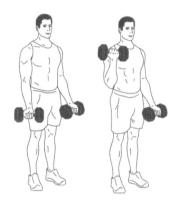

10 alt bicep curls
3 sets | 20 sec rest

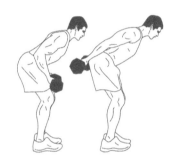

10 kickbacks
3 sets | 20 sec rest

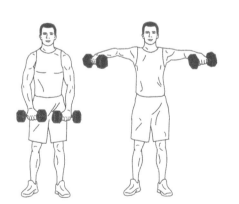

5 lateral raises
3 sets | 20 sec rest

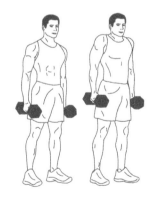

10 dumbbell shrugs
3 sets | 20 sec rest

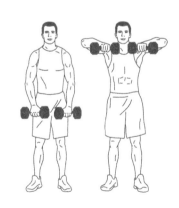

10 upright rows
3 sets | 20 sec rest

63 · Power 25

Resistance training with free weights can help increase upper body strength. Power 25 is a set routine you can use to push your upper body muscles into that performing zone that increases strength, activates muscle growth and helps develop power you can turn to functional strength.

Type: Classic
What It Works:

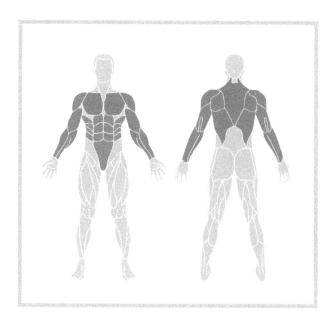

Power 25

DAREBEE WORKOUT © darebee.com

Use weights you can just do this routine with.
Pick up heavier weights the moment it gets easier.

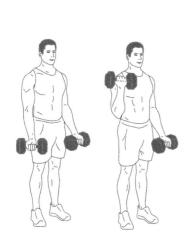

12 alt bicep curls
3 sets | 20 sec rest

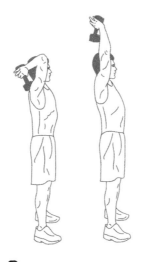

6 tricep extensions
3 sets | 20 sec rest

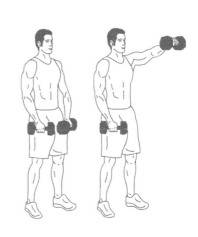

12 front arm raises
3 sets | 20 sec rest

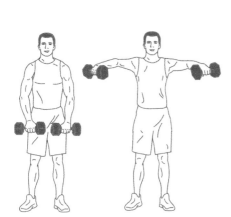

6 side arm raises
3 sets | 20 sec rest

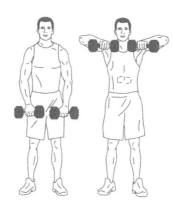

6 upright rows
3 sets | 20 sec rest

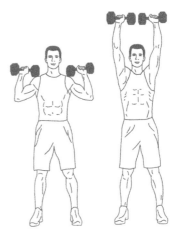

6 shoulder press
3 sets | 20 sec rest

64 Power Circuit Plus

Full body workouts recruit many different muscle groups for that holistic training experience. Power Circuit works all those muscles that need to be worked in order for your body to better utilize the strength it has and achieve higher power output at the physical performance level. The added weights only increase the muscle load you are applying.

Type: Circuit
What It Works:

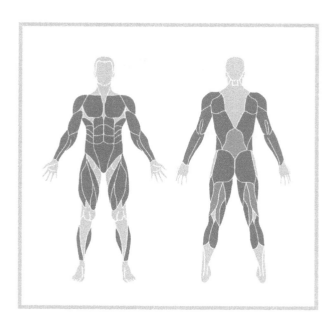

POWER CIRCUIT+

DAREBEE WORKOUT © darebee.com

LEVEL I 3 sets **LEVEL II** 5 sets **LEVEL III** 7 sets **REST** up to 2 minutes

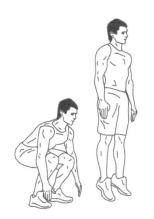

10 jump squats

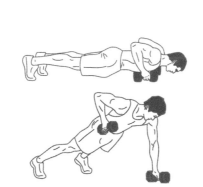

10 renegade row push-ups

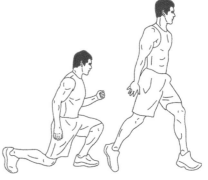

10 jumping lunges

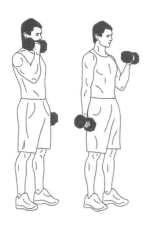

10 alt bicep curls

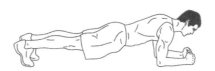

30sec elbow plank

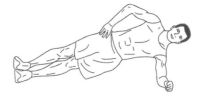

30sec side elbow plank

65 Power HIIT

The principle and benefits of High Intensity Interval Training (HIIT) can be applied to almost any physical activity, including the lifting of weights. Provided you have a couple of dumbbells that challenge you and a little time, you can make your body feel the need to change to meet the fresh demands being made upon it. This one not only gives you muscles that know the meaning of endurance but it also works on building strength.

Type: Circuit
What It Works:

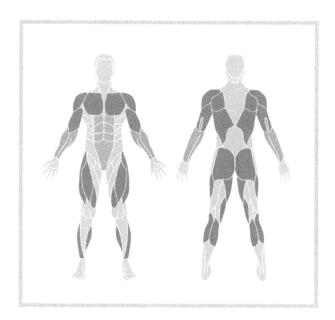

POWER

DAREBEE HIIT WORKOUT © darebee.com

LEVEL I 3 sets **LEVEL II** 5 sets **LEVEL III** 7 sets **REST** up to 2 minutes

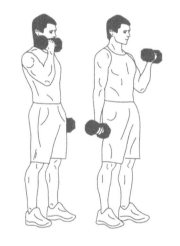

20sec alt bicep curls

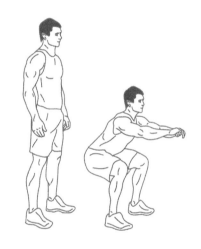

20sec squats

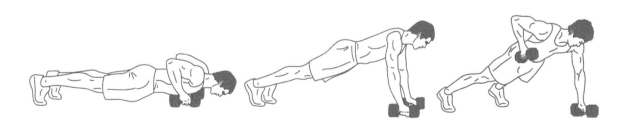

20sec renegade row push-ups

66 Power Pump

Power Pump helps you make excellent use of your dumbbells to build great upper body strength and muscle tone. If you have a set of dumbbells lurking around this is the perfect workout to use them in. Not only will it help you develop upper body strength but it is also great for maintaining core stability.

Type: Classic
What It Works:

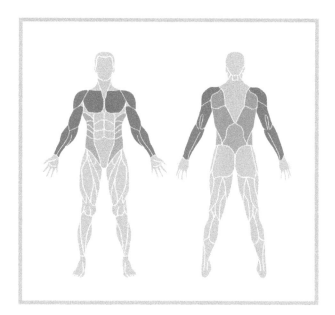

POWER PUMP

DAREBEE WORKOUT © darebee.com

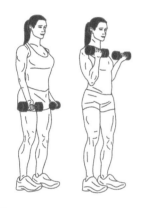

12 bicep curls x **5 sets**
60sec rest between sets

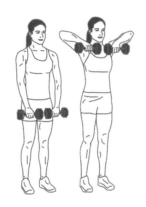

8 upright rows x **5 sets**
60sec rest between sets

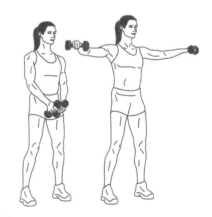

8 lateral raises x **5 sets**
60sec rest between sets

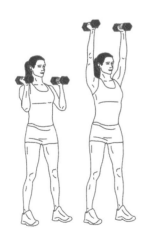

8 shoulder press x **5 sets**
60sec rest between sets

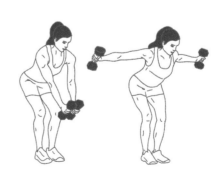

8 bent over raises x **5 sets**
60sec rest between sets

67. Power Row

If you have some dumbbells handy then add Power Row and you have yourself a total body strength workout that will make you feel like you've totally worked hard. Overall strength always helps improve athletic performance and with practically every muscle group targeted this is a program for building that overall strength you need to help boost your performance.

Type: Classic
What It Works:

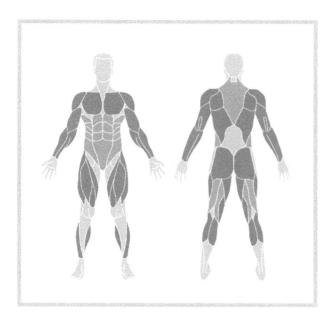

POWER ROW

DAREBEE
WORKOUT
© darebee.com

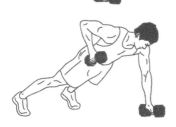

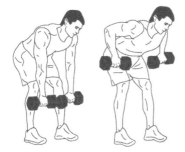

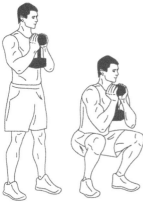

renegade rows
12, 10, 10, 8 (in total)
4 sets
20 seconds rest
between sets

bent over rows
10, 10, 8, 6
4 sets
20 seconds rest
between sets

goblet squats
12, 10, 10, 8
4 sets
20 seconds rest
between sets

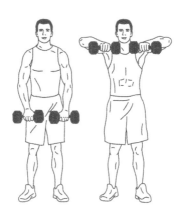

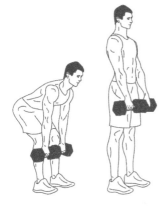

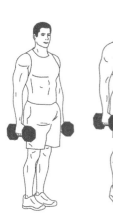

upright rows
10, 10, 8, 6
4 sets
20 seconds rest
between sets

deadlifts
8, 8, 6, 4
4 sets
20 seconds rest
between sets

calf raises
12, 10, 10, 8
4 sets
20 seconds rest
between sets

68 PPL Legs A

If you have a set of dumbbells the Push, Pull, Legs workout is the perfect means to build up strength and muscle. It's designed to trigger the adaptations the body needs to increase both muscle and strength and it recruits not just active muscles but also tendons and supporting muscle groups to give you a dynamic range of movement, under external, applied pressure. Combines with Push Pull Legs for upper body and Push Pull Legs for upper body and back.

Type: Classic
What It Works:

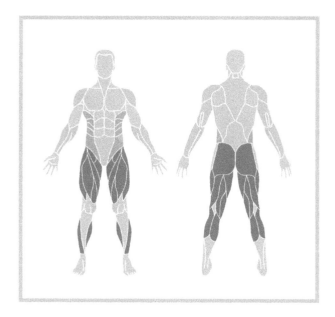

A PUSH PULL LEGS

2 minute rest between sets
2 minute rest between exercises
WORKOUT by
© darebee.com

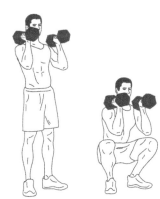

4 sets
squats
10-12 reps

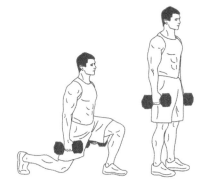

4 sets
reverse lunges
10-12 reps

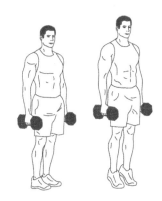

4 sets
calf raises
12-16 reps

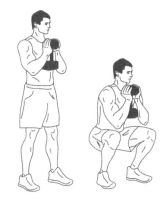

4 sets goblet squats
10-12 reps

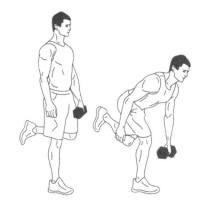

4 sets single leg deadlifts
5-6 reps / per side

69   PPL Legs B

Push, Pull, Legs B is an alternative to our Push Pull Legs A workout to provide you with a greater range of options for exercising your lower body. The workout build up lower body strength and muscle. It's designed to trigger the adaptations the body needs to increase both muscle and strength and it recruits not just active muscles but also tendons and supporting muscle groups to give you a dynamic range of movement, under external, applied pressure. Combines well with Push, Pull Legs for upper body and back and Push, Pull, Legs for upper body and abs for a complete set of Push, Pull, Legs workouts.

Type: Classic
What It Works:

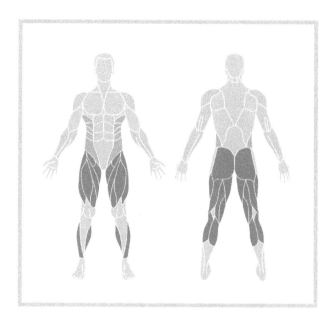

B PUSH PULL LEGS

2 minute rest between sets
2 minute rest between exercises
WORKOUT by
© darebee.com

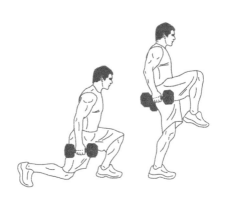

4 sets
lunge step-ups
10-12 reps

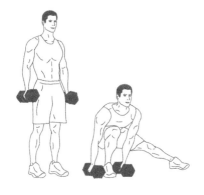

4 sets
side lunges
10-12 reps

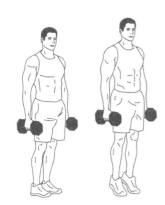

4 sets
calf raises
12-16 reps

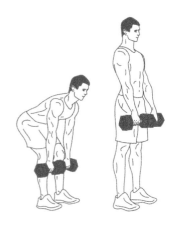

4 sets deadlifts
8-10 reps

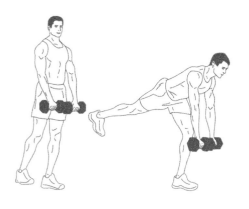

4 sets single leg deadlifts
5-6 reps / per side

70 PPL Pull A

This is perfect for the times you need an upper body Push, Pull, Legs workout. Combines well with Push Pull Legs workout for the lower body and Push Pull Legs for upper body and back to give you a set of exercises that target all the major muscle groups. Perfect for days when you want to focus on a particular body part and need to target those specific muscle groups.

Type: Classic
What It Works:

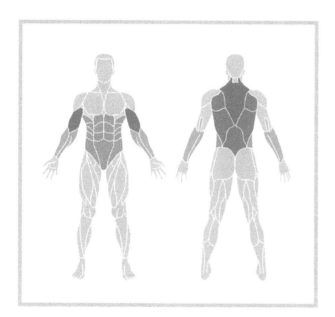

A PUSH PULL LEGS

2 minute rest between sets
2 minute rest between exercises
WORKOUT by
© darebee.com

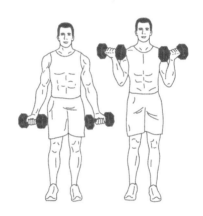

4 sets
bicep curls
8-12 reps

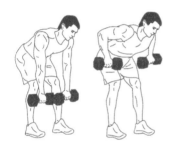

4 sets
bent over rows
8-10 reps

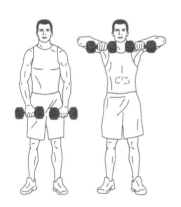

4 sets
upright rows
8-10 reps

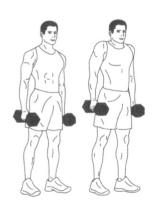

4 sets shrugs
8-10 reps

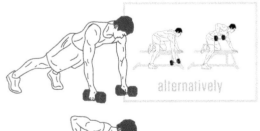

alternatively

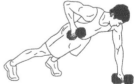

4 sets renegade rows
6-8 reps / per arm

71 PPL Pull B

Push, Pull, Legs workout for building upper body strength. It is an alternative to our Push, Pull, Legs workout. Perfect for days when you want to focus on a particular upper body part and need to target those specific muscle groups. It combines with Push, Pull, Legs for the lower body.

Type: Classic
What It Works:

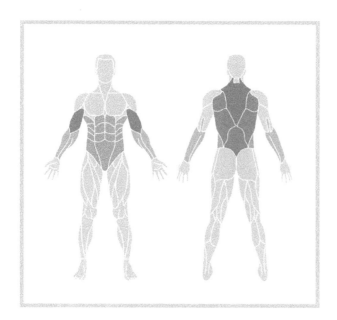

B PUSH PULL LEGS

2 minute rest between sets
2 minute rest between exercises
WORKOUT by
© darebee.com

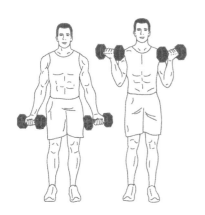

4 sets
bicep curls
8-12 reps

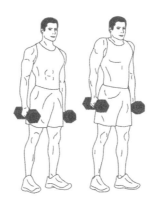

4 sets
shrugs
8-10 reps

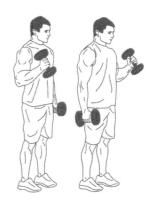

4 sets
hammer curls
10-12 reps

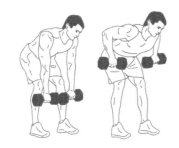

4 sets bent over rows
8-10 reps

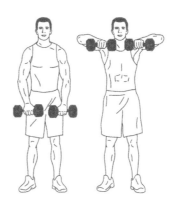

4 sets upright rows
8-10 reps

72

PPL Push A

This is a Push Pull Legs dumbbells workout that complements the Push Pull Legs for lower body and the Push Pull Legs upper body workout for a more rounded fitness routine. Put your dumbbells to great use by triggering the body's adaptation mechanism that helps you get fitter and stronger.

Type: Classic
What It Works:

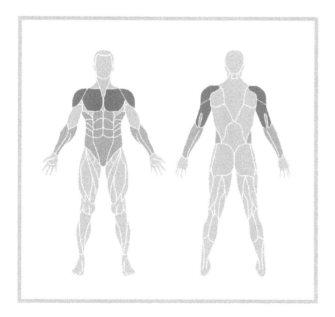

[A] PUSH PULL LEGS

2 minute rest between sets
2 minute rest between exercises
WORKOUT by
© darebee.com

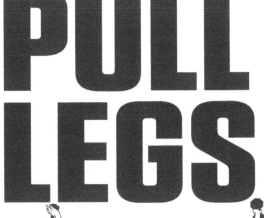

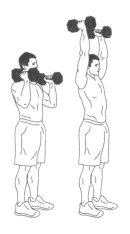

4 sets
shoulder press
6-10 reps

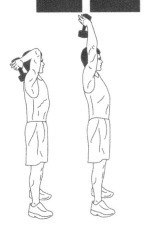

4 sets
overhead tricep extensions
5-7 reps / per arm

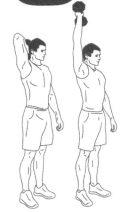

4 sets
tricep extensions
5-7 reps / per arm

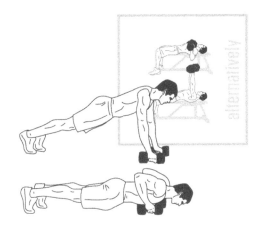

4 sets push-ups
10-14 reps

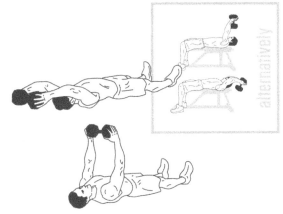

4 sets pullovers
6-10 reps

73

PPL Push B

Push, Pull, Legs B is an upper body and abs workout that is an alternative to Push, Pull Legs A for upper body and abs, It combines with Push, Pull, Legs B for lower body and Push, Pull, Legs B for upper body and back workout for a complete guide to a Push, Pull, Legs training plan.

Type: Classic
What It Works:

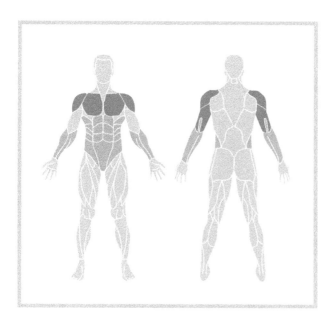

PUSH PULL LEGS

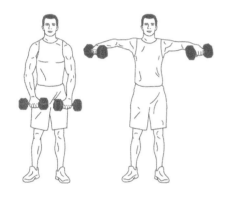

4 sets
lateral raises
6-10 reps

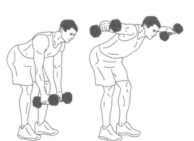

4 sets
bent over lateral raises
6-10 reps

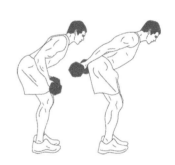

4 sets
tricep kickbacks
6-10 reps

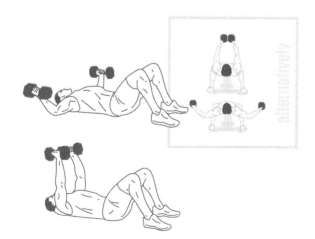

4 sets chest fly
8-10 reps

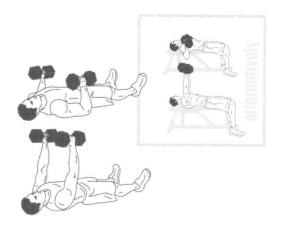

4 sets chest press
8-10 reps

74 Pure Power

If you have a good set of dumbbells you have the means to level up your strength through a full body, free weights workout. Pure Power works virtually every major muscle group.

Type: Classic
What It Works:

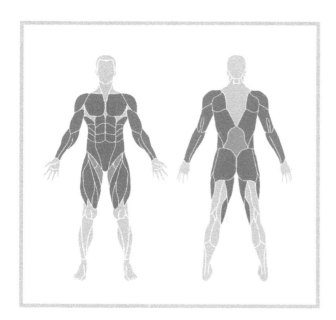

PURE POWER

DAREBEE WORKOUT © darebee.com

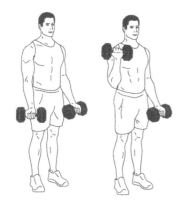

to fatigue bicep curls
3 sets | 20 seconds rest

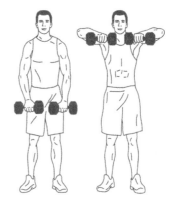

to fatigue upright rows
3 sets | 20 seconds rest

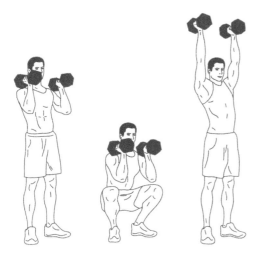

to fatigue squat into shoulder press
3 sets | 20 seconds rest

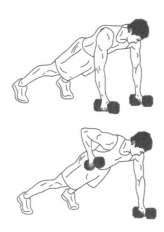

to fatigue renegade rows
3 sets | 20 seconds rest

75 Recomp

The Recomp is a full body strength workout that mixes bodyweight exercises and dumbbell ones to create a hybrid that pushes the muscles pretty hard. The result is a relentless load that just keeps on increasing forcing the body to activate the adaptation response necessary for strength gains.

Type: Circuit
What It Works:

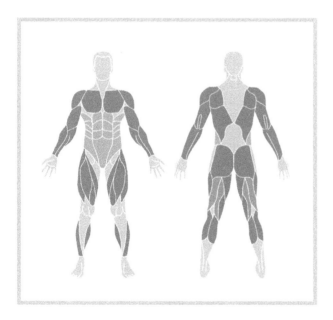

THE RECOMP

DAREBEE WORKOUT © darebee.com

LEVEL I 3 sets **LEVEL II** 5 sets **LEVEL III** 7 sets **REST** up to 2 minutes

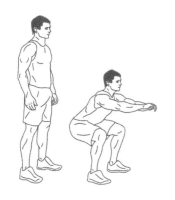

20 squats

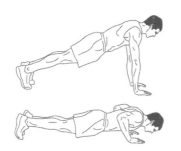

20 push-ups

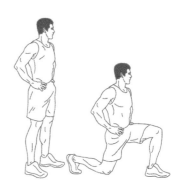

20 lunges

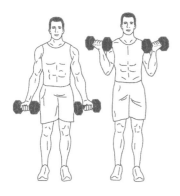

10 bicep curls

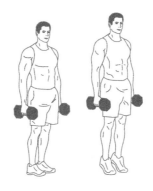

10 calf raises

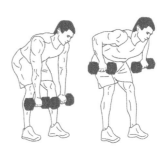

10 bent over rows

Renegade

If you're looking for an upper body workout that will make you feel the burn then The Renegade has to be your go-to workout. Form here is important. So is rest time between exercises.

Type: Classic
What It Works:

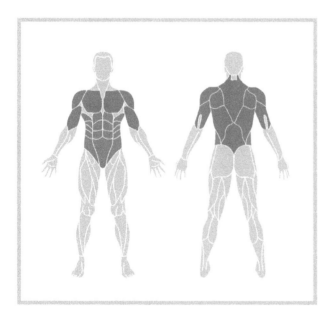

THE RENEGADE

DAREBEE WORKOUT © darebee.com

2 minutes rest between exercises

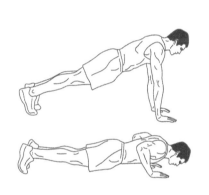

20 push-ups **x 4 sets** in total
20 seconds rest between sets

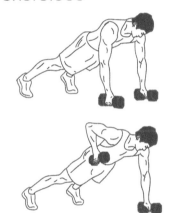

10 renegade rows **x 4 sets** in total
20 seconds rest between sets

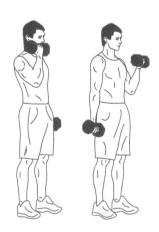

20 alt bicep curls **x 4 sets** in total
20 seconds rest between sets

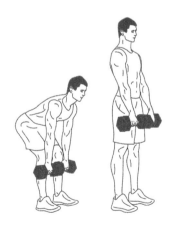

10 deadlifts **x 4 sets** in total
20 seconds rest between sets

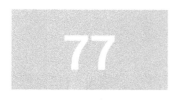 # Rise & Grind

Rise and Grind is a mix of bodyweight exercises and dumbbells to help you develop strength and tone. The mix is perfect for those who don't always want to use weights with the entire workout and there is a strong cardiovascular component to this workout that will also raise your body temperature.

Type: Classic
What It Works:

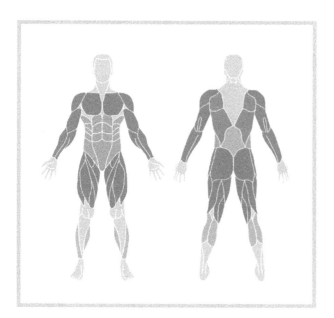

RISE AND GRIND

DAREBEE WORKOUT © darebee.com

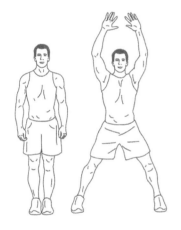

30 jumping jacks
4 sets in total
30 sec rest in between

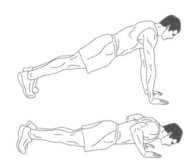

to fatigue push-ups
4 sets in total
30 sec rest in between

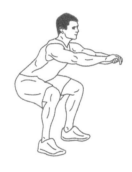

to fatigue squat hold
2 sets in total
30 sec rest in between

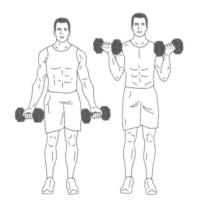

12 bicep curls
4 sets in total
30 sec rest in between

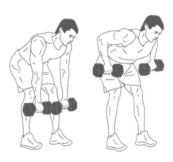

8 bent over rows
4 sets in total
30 sec rest in between

Sentinel Plus

Sentinel is a Level 4 total body strength workout. It's designed to push you into the sweat zone quickly and then keep you there as you go from one exercise to the next, working every major muscle group you have. It delivers strength, stability and an increased sense of power. Increase the push-up count for EC and you also feel the burn in your arms, shoulders and chest.

Type: Circuit
What It Works:

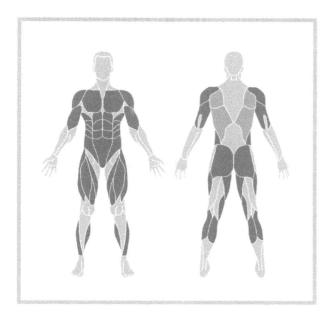

SENTINEL+

DAREBEE WORKOUT © darebee.com

LEVEL I 3 sets **LEVEL II** 5 sets **LEVEL III** 7 sets **REST** up to 2 minutes

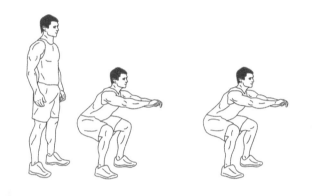

4combos: **10** squats + **10-count** hold

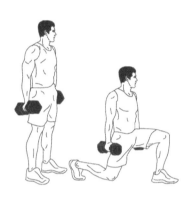

20 lunges

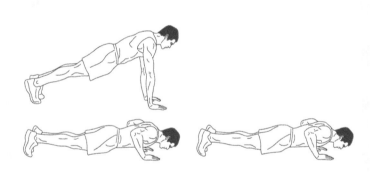

4combos: **5** push-ups + **5-count** hold

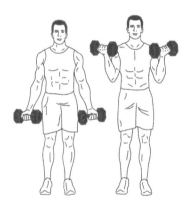

20 bicep curls

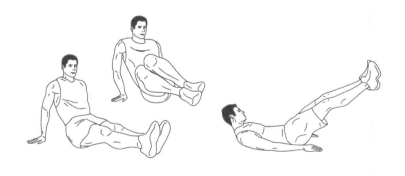

4combos: **10** knee-in & twist + **10-count** hold

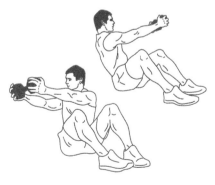

20 sitting twists

79 Serious Lifts

If you have a set of barbells you are ready to experience the workout called Serious Lifts. An upper body workout designed to take you to the limit of your ability Serious Lifts is designed to help you get stronger and build the kind of quality muscle that makes you feel like you can do almost anything.

Type: Classic
What It Works:

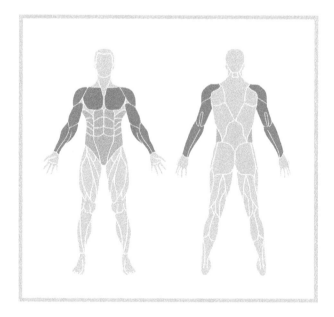

SERIOUS LIFTS

DAREBEE WORKOUT © darebee.com

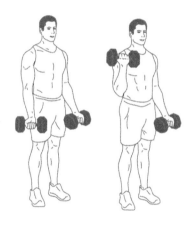

to fatigue alternating bicep curls
x 5 sets in total | 20 seconds rest

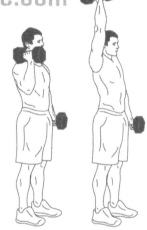

to fatigue alternating shoulder press
x 5 sets in total | 20 seconds rest

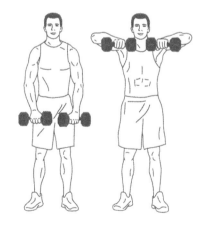

to fatigue upright rows
x 5 sets in total | 20 seconds rest

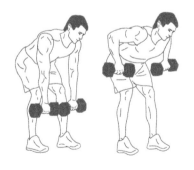

to fatigue bent over rows
x 5 sets in total | 20 seconds rest

80 Shredder Plus

The Shredder workout lets you remake your body by focusing on strength building in a dynamic, flowing way. It targets the body's major muscle groups building up the pressure as muscles fatigue. When it comes to conditioning this is a workout that can truly deliver the goods. Executed while keeping perfect form delivers some incredible gains in strength.

Type: Circuit
What It Works:

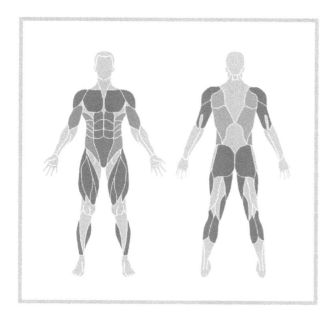

SHREDDER+

DAREBEE WORKOUT © darebee.com

LEVEL I 3 sets **LEVEL II** 5 sets **LEVEL III** 7 sets **REST** up to 2 minutes

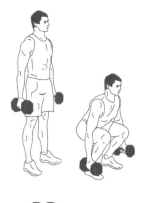

20 squats

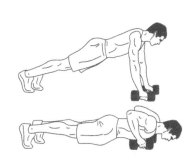

10 push-ups

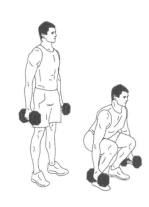

20 squats

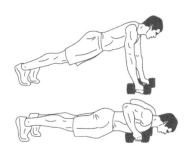

10 push-ups

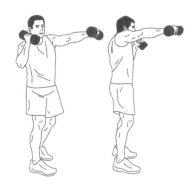

20 punches

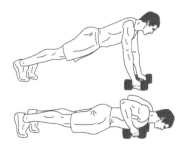

10 push-ups

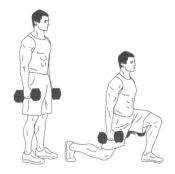

20 lunges

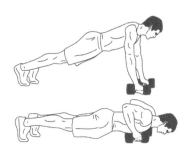

10 push-ups

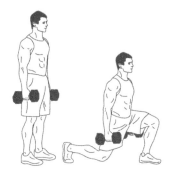

20 lunges

81 Smiter

Make your upper body weep with the The Smiter workout. Specifically designed to transform you into a formidable striking machine it gives your upper body muscles barely a breather as it takes you from one exercise to the next. A couple of things to watch on form here: A. When your body's straight keep your abs slightly tensed and do not lean forward when lifting, that way you work abs, core and lower back. B. When doing shoulder press always bring the weight to balance first at the very top of the shoulder (without touching), that way; when you lift you also activate the upper back muscles. C. Watch the grip changes in the shoulder press between the first and last rows of exercises, they activate different muscles groups and spread the load differently.

Type: Classic   **What It Works:**

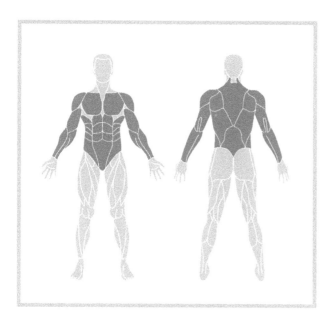

THE SMITER

DAREBEE WORKOUT © darebee.com
2 minutes rest between combos and sets

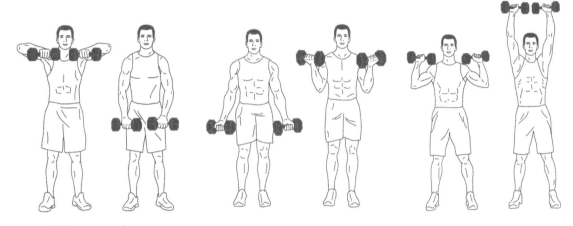

10combos upright row + bicep curl -+ shoulder press **x 3 sets**

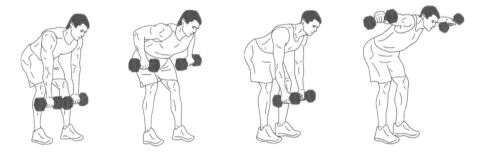

10combos bent over row + bent over lateral raise **x 3 sets**

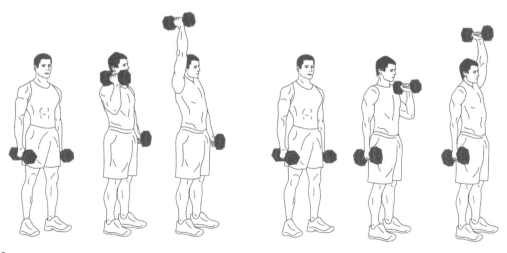

10combos hammer curl, right + shoulder press + hammer curl, left + shoulder press **x 3 sets**

82 Steelworks Plus

Steelworks Plus is a combat mode workout that utilizes weights to deliver a targeted load to your muscles. The workout takes your body and puts it through a series of combat moves that recruit almost every major muscle group. It pushes your endurance. It challenges muscle recovery. It's great for your balance. It requires speed and precision and it challenges your VO2 Max too.

Type: Circuit
What It Works:

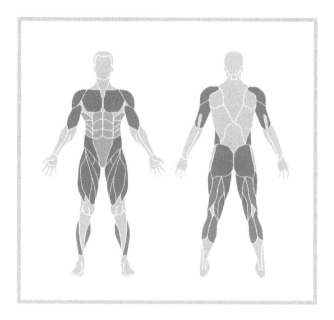

STEEL WORKS+

DAREBEE WORKOUT © darebee.com

LEVEL I 3 sets **LEVEL II** 5 sets **LEVEL III** 7 sets **REST** up to 2 minutes

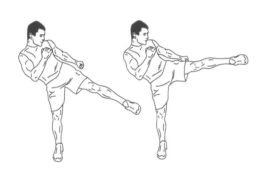

20 double turning kicks

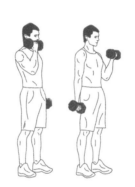

20 alt bicep curls

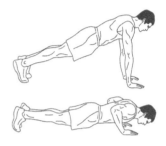

10 push-ups

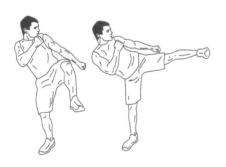

20 side kicks

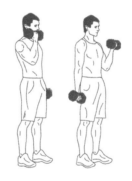

20 alt bicep curls

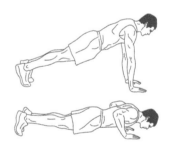

10 push-ups

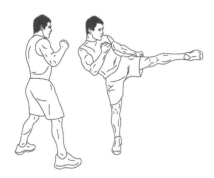

20 back leg tunring kicks

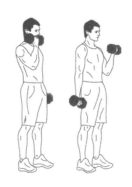

20 alt bicep curls

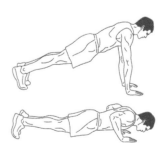

10 push-ups

83 Strength & Power

Upper body strength is hard to build. It requires many different muscles groups to feel sufficient load to trigger the body's adaptive response. And it needs those muscle groups to recruit additional muscle groups and work in a both concentric and eccentric fashion in order to build up power. The Strength & Power workout does all this.

Type: Classic
What It Works:

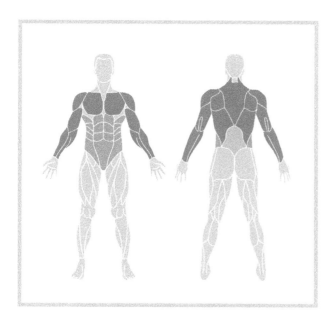

STRENGTH & POWER

DAREBEE WORKOUT © darebee.com

2 minutes rest between exercises

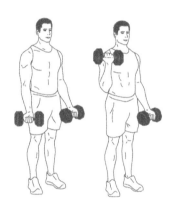

20 alternating
bicep curls
x 3 sets in total
20 seconds rest
between sets

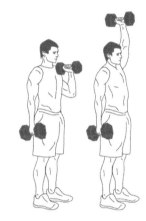

20 alternating
shoulder press
x 3 sets in total
20 seconds rest
between sets

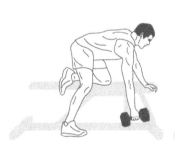
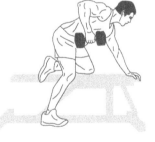

20 bent over rows **x 3 sets** in total
20 seconds rest between sets

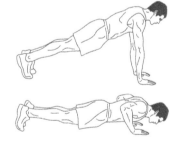

20 push-ups **x 3 sets** in total
20 seconds rest between sets

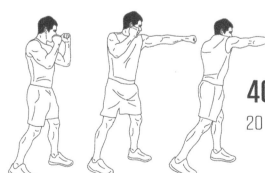

40 punches **x 3 sets** in total
20 seconds rest between sets

84 Strong & Beautiful

An upper body strength and tone workout that helps you improve the way your upper body works can only be called Strong & Beautiful. A series of consecutive exercises load your muscles and recruit upper body tendons to help you build a sense of power and control.

Type: Circuit
What It Works:

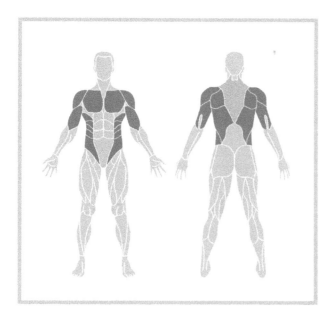

STRONG & BEAUTIFUL

DAREBEE WORKOUT © darebee.com

LEVEL I 3 sets   **LEVEL II** 4 sets   **LEVEL III** 5 sets   **REST** up to 2 minutes

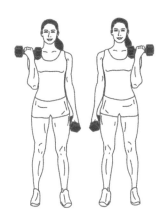

20 alt bicep curls

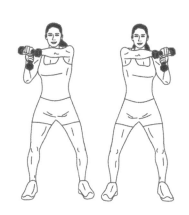

20 punches

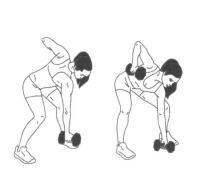

10 bent over rows

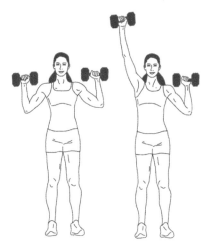

10 alt shoulder press

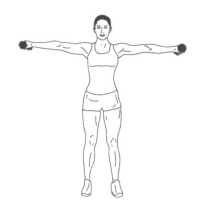

10-count hold

Stuntman

Stuntman is a full-body, explore-the-limits of your ability strength workout. It tasks virtually every part of your body so it will, also, challenge your cardiovascular system. The difficulty level of this workout makes it unsuitable for beginners but it does give you a target to keep on your radar for the future as you progress along your fitness journey.

Type: Circuit
What It Works:

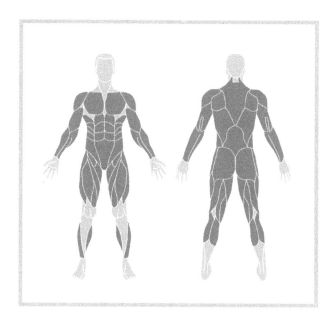

STUNTMAN

DAREBEE WORKOUT © darebee.com

LEVEL I 3 sets **LEVEL II** 4 sets **LEVEL III** 5 sets **REST** up to 2 minutes

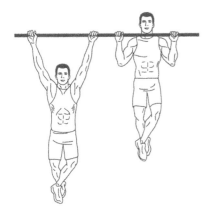

max pull-ups

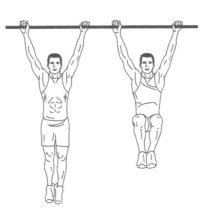

max knee-ins

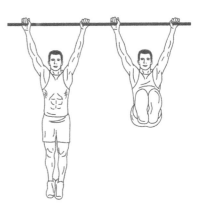

max leg raises

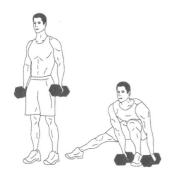

12 side lunges

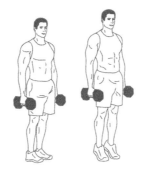

12 calf raises

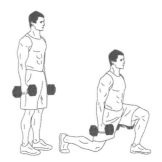

12 lunges

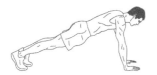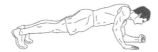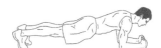

12 up & down planks

86 Superhero Strength Plus

Superheroes move and function like gravity doesn't exist. They use their body like it has no mass but punch and kick with immense power. The Superhero Strength Plus workout uses weights and bodyweight exercises to hyperload the body's muscle groups triggering the adaptive response and helping you develop the kind of strength and power the super hero in you demands to have.

Type: Classic
What It Works:

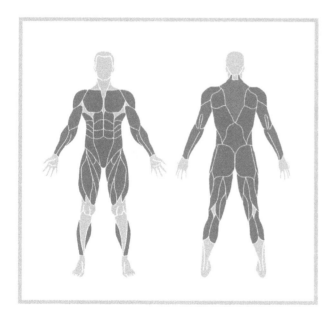

superhero strength PLUS

DAREBEE
WORKOUT
© darebee.com

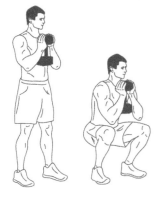

20 goblet squats
5 sets in total
30 seconds rest

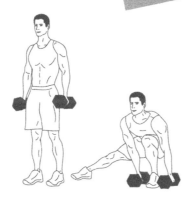

20 side lunges
5 sets in total
30 seconds rest

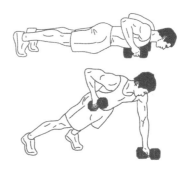

20 renegade row push-ups
5 sets in total
30 seconds rest

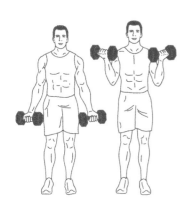

20 bicep curls
5 sets in total
30 seconds rest

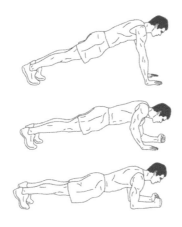

20 up & down planks
5 sets in total
30 seconds rest

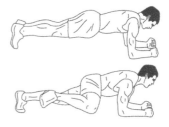

20 elbow plank
side crunches
5 sets in total
30 seconds rest

87 Super Strength

Dumbbells add an external load on the body that is immutable. As muscles tire and the load doesn't ease they degrade. The damage they sustain triggers the body's adaptive response and muscle protein synthesis kicks in to repair muscle tissue that has sustained damage due to exercise-induced stress and help it become stronger and larger. Super Strength is a strength-building workout designed specifically to help you achieve your strength goals.

Type: Classic
What It Works:

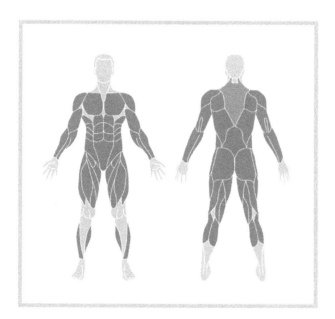

SUPER STRENGTH

DAREBEE WORKOUT © darebee.com

20 seconds rest between sets | 20 seconds rest between exercises

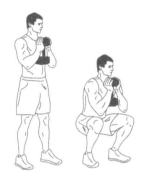

10 goblet squats
x 3 sets

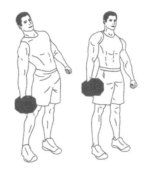

10 side bends
x 3 sets

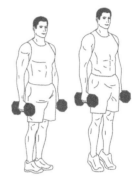

10 calf raises
x 3 sets

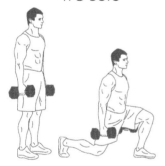

10 forward lunges
x 3 sets

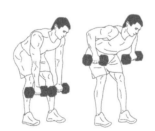

10 bent over rows
x 3 sets

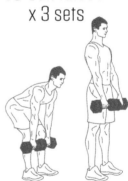

10 deadlifts
x 3 sets

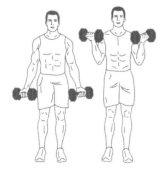

10 bicep curls
x 3 sets

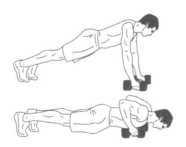

10 push-ups
x 3 sets

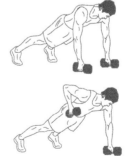

10 renegade rows
x 3 sets

Threshold

Threshold is a strength and muscle building workout. It requires dumbbells and good form. Pay attention to the speed of execution of each movement and slow them down as much as you can in order to recruit more muscle fibers and activate more adaptations that will lead to stronger muscles and bones.

Type: Circuit
What It Works:

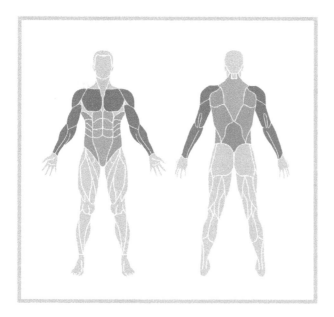

THRESHOLD

DAREBEE WORKOUT © darebee.com

LEVEL I 3 sets **LEVEL II** 4 sets **LEVEL III** 5 sets **REST** up to 2 minutes

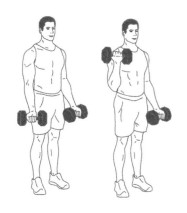

12 alt bicep curls

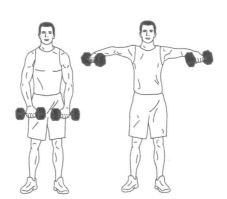

12 lateral raises

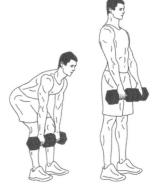

12 deadlifts

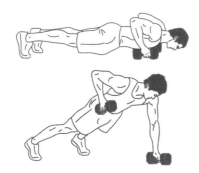

12 push-up renegade rows

89 Trim & Tone Arms

Muscles are taut and strong. They make your body yours to control and trivialize gravity by either giving you the ability to move your body like it is lighter or lift heavy stuff like its mass doesn't matter. The Trim & Tone workout targets the upper body focusing on the arms and shoulders for that battle-ready look of streamlined muscles, ready to be put to good work.

Type: Classic
What It Works:

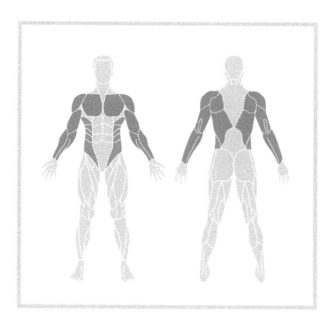

TRIM & TONE ARMS

WORKOUT
by DAREBEE
© darebee.com
2 minutes rest
between exercises

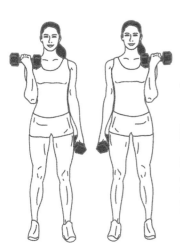

12 reps
5 sets
alternating bicep curls
20 seconds rest
between sets

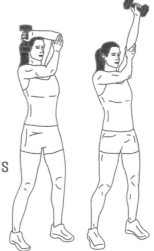

12 reps
5 sets
tricep extensions
20 seconds rest
between sets

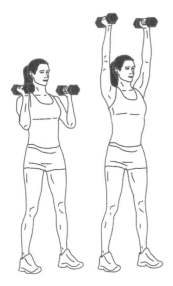

6 reps
5 sets
shoulder press
20 seconds rest
between sets

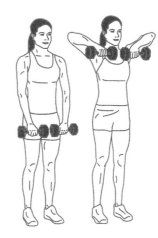

6 reps
5 sets
body rows
20 seconds rest
between sets

90 Tyr

Tyr is a workout that's designed to put the dumbbells you have to really good use. This means you will feel the load and that sensation will trigger the adaptation response you need. While this targets the lower body, studies show that it also, in small ways, affects the upper body.

Type: Classic
What It Works:

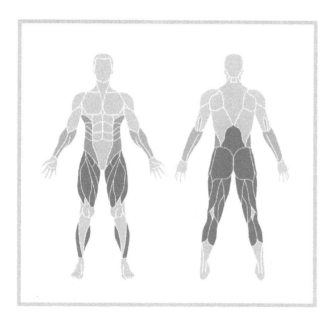

TYR

DAREBEE WORKOUT © darebee.com

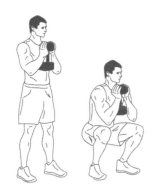

12 goblet squats
5 sets in total
30 sec rest in between

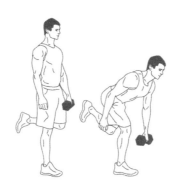

12 single leg deadlifts
5 sets in total
30 sec rest in between

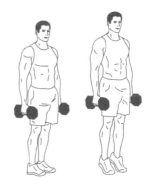

12 calf raises
5 sets in total
30 sec rest in between

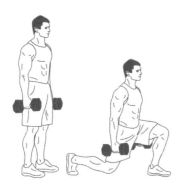

12 lunges
5 sets in total
30 sec rest in between

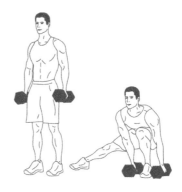

12 side lunges
5 sets in total
30 sec rest in between

91   Under Construction

The body is a construct. It is the result of genetics and environment, nutrition and biochemistry. Part of it we inherit. Some of it is the result of how and where we grew up. But some of it is ours to build and own. We have the ability to construct the body we want to live in and its capabilities. The Under Construction Workout is an equipment-based workout that requires you to have a set of dumbbells and some time. The way you will feel after it is over will be totally worth it.

Type: Classic
What It Works:

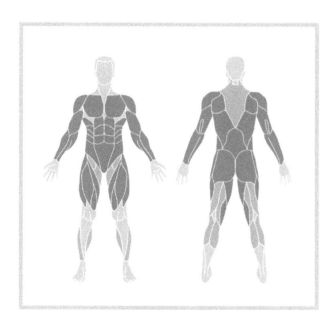

UNDER CONSTRUCTION

DAREBEE WORKOUT © darebee.com

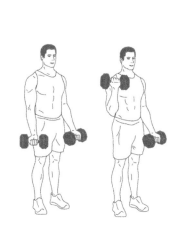

20 bicep curls
4 sets in total
30 sec rest in between

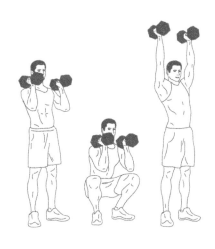

10 squat into press
4 sets in total
30 sec rest in between

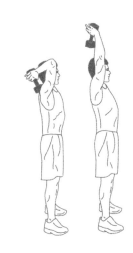

10 tricep extensions
4 sets in total
30 sec rest in between

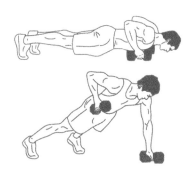

to fatigue push-up renegade rows
4 sets in total
30 sec rest in between

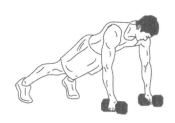

30 seconds plank hold
2 sets in total
30 sec rest in between

92 Upperbody Blast

Blast your upper body strength to a new level with the Upper Body Blast workout. You need some dumbbells. A little bit of time and the key ingredient supplied by a body ready to be strength-trained and you have yourself everything required for a transformational experience.

Type: Classic
What It Works:

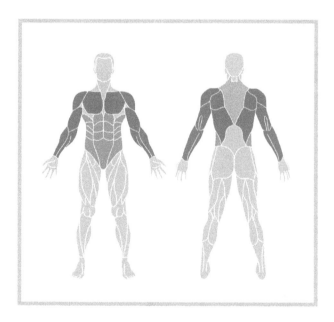

UPPERBODY BLAST

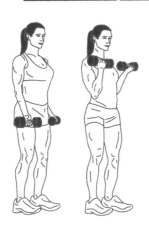

8 bicep curl
x 3 sets in total
20 seconds rest
between sets

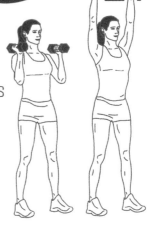

8 shoulder press
x 3 sets in total
20 seconds rest
between sets

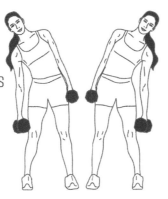

8 side-to-side tilts
x 3 sets in total
20 seconds rest
between sets

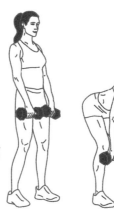

8 deadlifts
x 3 sets in total
20 seconds rest
between sets

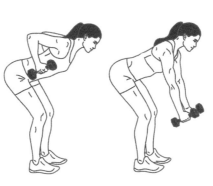

8 bent over rows
x 3 sets in total
20 seconds rest
between sets

93 Upperbody Builder

Circuit training with weights is probably one of the hardest things you can do. Muscles get tired quickly and because of the added extraneous load they do not recover that fast, which means you go into the next set already fatigued. Upperbody Builder helps you build up strength on your upper body.

Type: Circuit
What It Works:

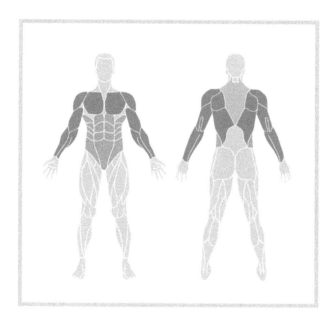

UPPERBODY BUILDER

MUSCLE BUILDING WORKOUT BY DAREBEE © darebee.com

Repeat one exercise after the other with no rest in between.

3 sets - 2 minutes rest between sets

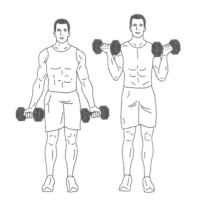

10 bicep curls

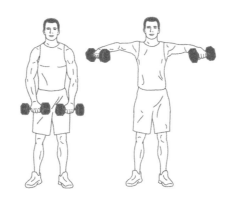

5 lateral raises

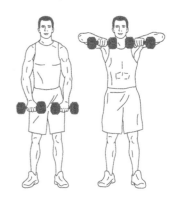

5 chest rows

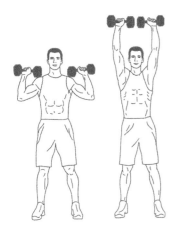

5 shoulder press

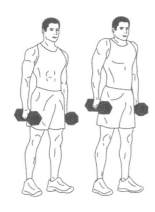

5 shrugs

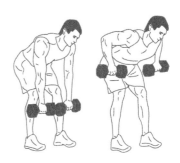

5 bent over rows

Upperbody Forge

Resistance work with extra weight amplifies the forces applied to the muscles and accelerates the body's adaptive response. As a result strength gains are accelerated and the body's muscles become stronger and denser. The Upperbody Forge is a workout that truly lives up to its name with a set of exercises targeting all major upper body muscle groups. Great if you have a couple of dumbbells lying around and feel like doing some muscle-sculpting work.

Type: Classic
What It Works:

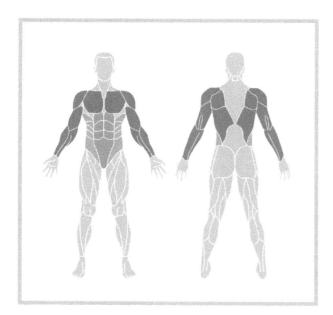

UPPERBODY
FORGE

DAREBEE WORKOUT © darebee.com

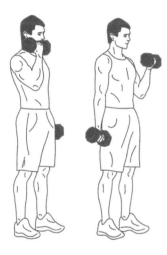

10 bicep curls
x 4 sets in total

20 seconds rest
between sets

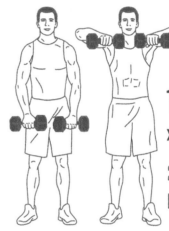

10 upright rows
x 4 sets in total

20 seconds rest
between sets

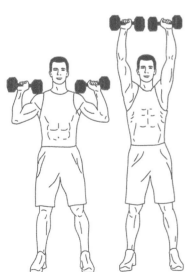

10 shoulder press
x 4 sets in total

20 seconds rest
between sets

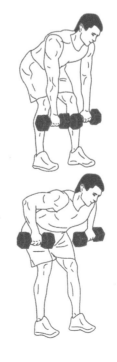

10 bent over rows
x 4 sets in total

20 seconds rest
between sets

95 Upperbody Tendon Strength Plus

The Upper Body Tendon Strength Plus workout delivers the best results when you perform slow, precise movements, tighten your abs to stabilize your body and make sure you pivot correctly off your feet with each punch. Use 1-3kg (2-6lb) dumbbells for this workout. Don't forget to breathe.

Type: Classic
What It Works:

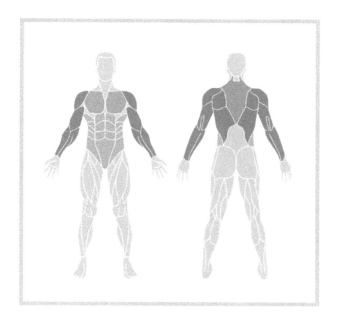

UPPERBODY
TENDON
STRENGTH+

DAREBEE WORKOUT © darebee.com

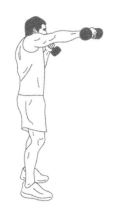

30sec dumbbell hold
right arm

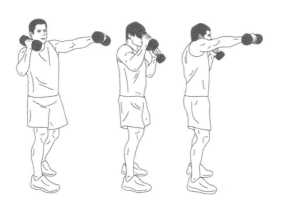

10sec punches
slow motion

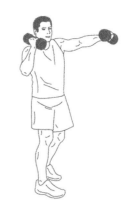

30sec dumbbell hold
left arm

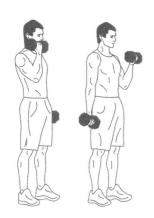

30sec bicep curls
slow motion

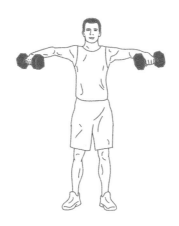

10sec hold

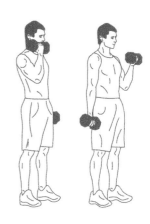

30sec bicep curls
slow motion

Upper Body Sculpt

We may have once lived in trees but since then we've lost all the upper body strength that helped keep us safe. This is a workout designed to address our deficiencies in that department. It may not quite make us capable of reclaiming our arboreal environment but at least the Upper Body Sculpt will make us feel like we could.

Type: Classic
What It Works:

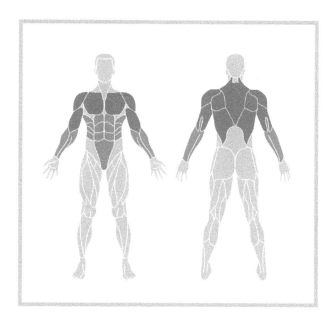

UPPER BODY
SCULPT

WORKOUT BY
© darebee.com

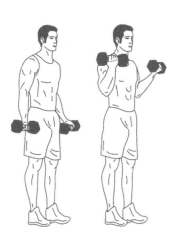

bicep curls
12, 10, 8, 6
20 seconds rest

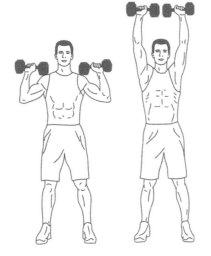

shoulder press
12, 10, 8, 6
20 seconds rest

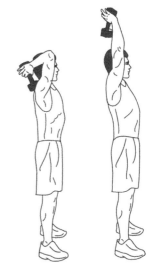

tricep extensions
9, 7, 5, 3
20 seconds rest

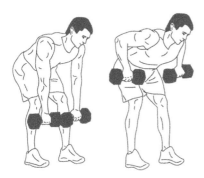

bent over rows
10, 8, 6, 4
20 seconds rest

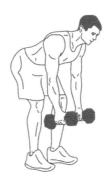

bent over raises
10, 8, 6, 4
20 seconds rest

97 Valour

If you have some dumbbells now's the time to reach for them. Valour is a dumbbell workout that will help your muscles get stronger and your body leaner. Because it's an additional load to the body you need to maintain perfect form and slow down your repetitions so you can engage more muscles.

Type: Classic
What It Works:

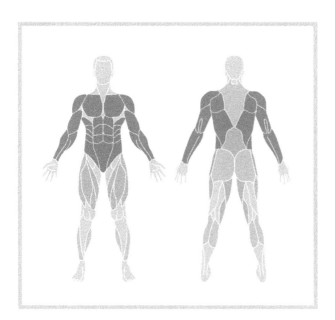

VALOUR

DAREBEE WORKOUT © darebee.com

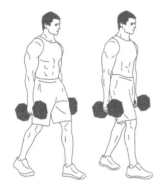

60 seconds farmer's walk
3 sets in total
60 sec rest in between

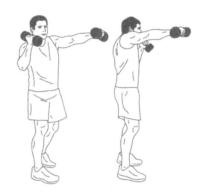

60 seconds punches
3 sets in total
60 sec rest in between

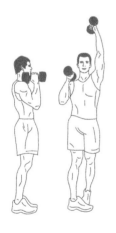

30 seconds

overhead punches
3 sets in total
60 sec rest in between

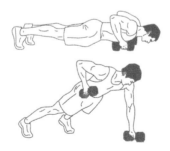

30 seconds

renegade rows
3 sets in total
60 sec rest in between

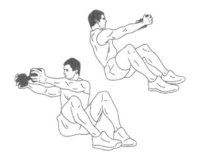

30 seconds

sitting twists
3 sets in total
60 sec rest in between

98   V-Taper

Shape your upper body with the V-Taper Workout. Focus on form and go as slow and possible. Make sure you clear the bar and then slowly lower yourself down when performing pull-ups. Use a wider grip if possible. If you find bent over raises too difficult to perform with heavier weights, use lighter ones but, again, lift and then lower them as slow as possible.

Type: Classic
What It Works:

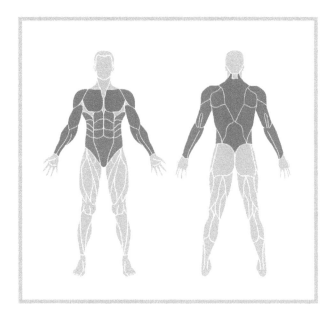

V taper

DAREBEE WORKOUT © darebee.com
2 minutes rest between exercises

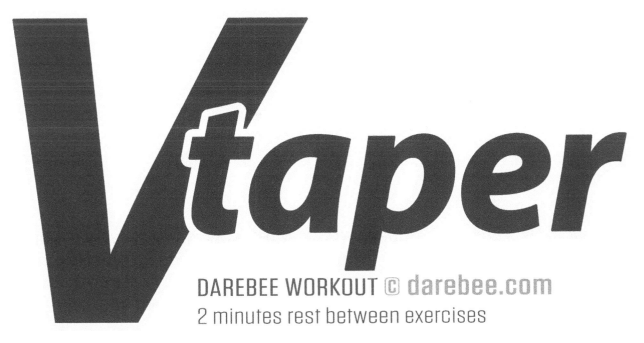

to failure pull-ups
5 sets in total | 20 seconds rest

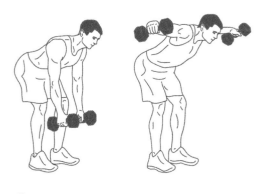

8 bent over raises **x 5 sets** in total
20 seconds rest between sets

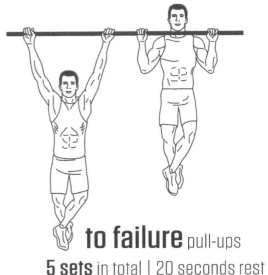

8 kneeling rows **x 5 sets** in total
20 seconds rest between sets

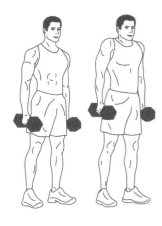

8 shrugs **x 5 sets** in total
20 seconds rest between sets

99 Work Of Art

Work Of Art is a dumbbells-based workout that works almost every major muscle group in the body enhancing strength and developing muscle tone. Perfect for the days when you can't run outside because it's too cold, too dark or too wet but still need to feel you're not losing ground.

Type: Circuit
What It Works:

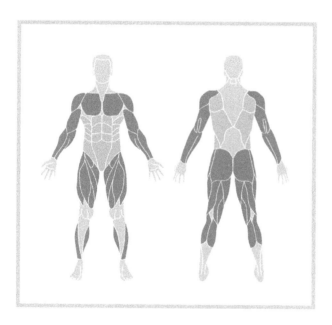

WORK OF ART

DAREBEE WORKOUT © darebee.com

LEVEL I 3 sets **LEVEL II** 5 sets **LEVEL III** 7 sets **REST** up to 2 minutes

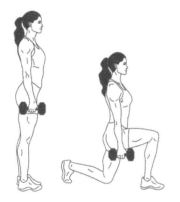

12 lunges

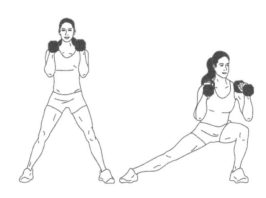

8 side lunges

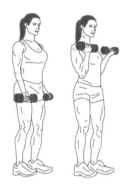

12 bicep curls

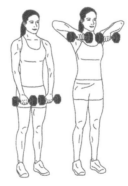

8 upright rows

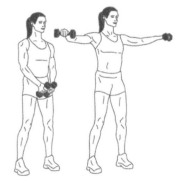

8 lateral raises

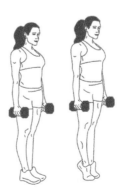

12 calf raises

100   XXL Biceps

Size is not the only component of strength but, in general, bigger muscles lead to strength gains. This is where XXL Biceps comes in. A workout where form is important and speed of execution of each has to be as slow as possible in order to recruit as many muscle fibers as possible. Choose a weight that is challenging and maintain a tight core throughout by positioning your body properly to engage it.

Type: Classic
What It Works:

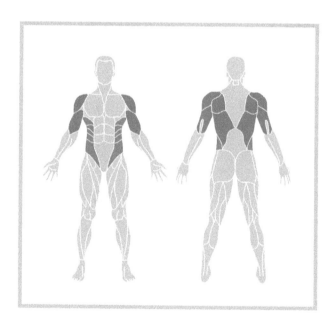

XXL BICEPS

DAREBEE WORKOUT © darebee.com

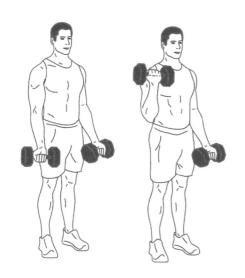

to failure alternating bicep curls

2 minutes rest

to failure alternating bicep curls

2 minutes rest

to failure alternating bicep curls

2 minutes rest

to failure bent over rows, right side

to failure bent over rows, left side

2 minutes rest

to failure bent over rows, right side

to failure bent over rows, left side

2 minutes rest

to failure bent over rows, right side

to failure bent over rows, left side

done

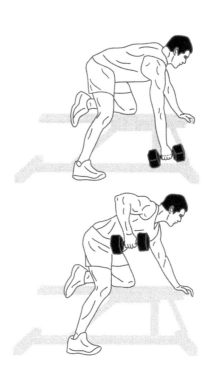

Immerse Your Mind and Change Your Body

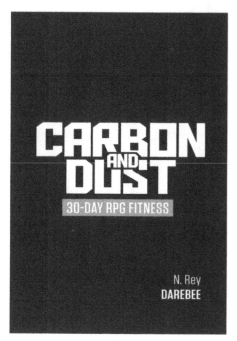

Carbon & Dust is a 30-day Darebee Role Playing Game (RPG), fitness action-adventure with you as the main protagonist. It is set in a distant future when humanity has spread far and wide across the Galaxy. It's a world where the corporations set and keep the laws and where you can only rely on your own strength, speed and cunning.

To survive, you must become a weapon. To make a difference, you must be prepared to give it your all. To win and stay alive you must be prepared to push past your limits.

This program can be completed one chapter per day (recommended). The program reads like a book with integrated action and tasks you must complete to advance further in the story. Through the exercises and workouts you get to develop balance and coordination, speed and endurance, strength and power.

Like every RPG fitness action-adventure this one holds the power to transform your mind as well as your body. You will find yourself having to make moral choices and back them up with physical action. You will balance the need for survival against what you feel is the right thing to do.

Every choice will cost you. Every decision will take you deeper into a world where you get to decide how the struggle to maintain the balance in the universe unfolds.

Enter the world of Carbon and Dust and see just how far it'll take you.

Unleash Your Inner Hero!

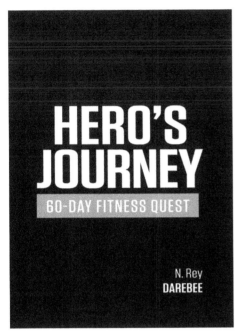

Hero's Journey is a role-playing fitness program inspired by every hero's transformation from minion to master.

Each day takes you through a stage of the journey, presents you with fresh challenges, opportunities and threats. Each of these is accompanied by exercises that test your skill, push your performance and require you to adapt and develop in order to go on. The role play scenario transports your mind into situations where you face incredible odds and have to fight to survive. In the process you get to change not just physically but also mentally.

The routines are designed to immerse you into imaginative scenarios where you have to push your mind, forcing yourself to dig deep to find the willpower to not give up, fight the good fight and come out the other side. The journey is 60 days long and it is totally transformative.

When you have really traveled the hero's path and have gone through your quest, you will have shed uncertainty, fear and doubt along with excess body weight. You will have forged a new character out of yourself, build strength and endurance and developed power. You will stand confident in who you are and what you can do: a true hero to yourself.

Page left blank intentionally